IN SEARCH OF MANHOOD

Problems, causes and solutions

PETER DORNAN

Published in Australia by Sid Harta Books & Print Pty Ltd,
ABN: 34632585293
23 Stirling Crescent, Glen Waverley, Victoria 3150 Australia
Telephone: +61 3 9560 9920, Facsimile: +61 3 9545 1742
E-mail: author@sidharta.com.au

First published in Australia 2024
This edition published 2024
Copyright © Peter Dornan 2024
Cover design, typesetting: WorkingType (www.workingtype.com.au)

The right of Peter Dornan to be identified as the
Author of the Work has been asserted in accordance with the
Copyright, Designs and Patents Act 1988.

All rights reserved. No part of this publication may be reproduced, stored in a retrieval system, or transmitted, in any form or by any means without the prior written permission of the publisher, nor be otherwise circulated in any form of binding or cover other than that in which it is published and without a similar condition being imposed on the subsequent purchaser.

ISBN: 978-1-922958-81-5

About the Author

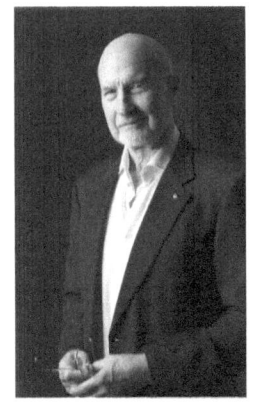

For fifty-seven years, Peter Dornan has been a physiotherapist in the fields of sports medicine and manipulative therapy. He has worked with many international sporting teams, including being the inaugural physiotherapist for the Australian national rugby union team, the Australian national rugby league team, the Queensland rugby union team, and the Australian cricket team.

For his achievements, he was awarded the Commemorative 2000 Australian Sports Medal. He is also a passionate men's health activist. In 1997, Peter created a forum for men and their partners to gain support and be better informed in matters relating to prostate cancer. He was influential in forming the Prostate Cancer Foundation of Australia.

Peter has been freelance writing for many years and written two books on sporting injuries, one on prostate cancer (*Conquering Incontinence*), two on pelvic pain, and four military books (*The Silent Men*, an account of the Kokoda Track campaign, *Nicky Barr – An Australian Air Ace*, *The Last Man Standing*, an account of the Tobruk and El Alamein campaigns, and *Diving Stations,* an inspiring story of one of the most successful submarine commanders of the Second World War). In 2002, Peter was appointed a member of the General Division of the Order of Australia (AM) and was the 2020 Queensland Senior Australian of the Year.

Peter has been a classical sculptor for more than forty years with works in many national institutions and private collections.

Peter is married to Dr Dimity Dornan (AO), a speech pathologist, who is the founder and director of Hear and Say, a world-wide charity which teaches babies who are deaf to listen and to speak. She is also the founder and chair of Bionics Queensland and Bionics Gamechangers Australia. They have two adult children, Melissa and Roderick.

Further information: **www.peterdornanphysio.com.au**

Other titles by Peter Dornan

Conquering Incontinence

So you've got Pelvic Pain…here's how to manage it

The Silent Men – an account of the Kokoda Track Campaign

Nicky Barr – An Australian Air Ace

The Last Man Standing,

Diving Stations

DEDICATION

This book is dedicated to my good friend and bon vivant, the ever erudite, Emeritus Professor Bob Milns AM. Bob was Professor of Classics and Ancient History at the University of Queensland for a record thirty-three years (1970-2003).

He was an enduring source of great inspiration for many of my mythological and classical sculpture and writing projects. We shared a love of history, music, singing and whistling, while gathering completely useless information over a good red.

Bob died of complications from myeloma and prostate cancer in 2020, at the age of eighty-two.

ACKNOWLEDGMENTS

To write a book of this nature is one that I could not attempt alone. I have relied on many personal interviews, anecdotes and stories freely shared by a great number of men and their partners.

I have accessed relevant books, research journals and popular press articles focussing on various aspects of these themes, generally acknowledging their authority in the text. In particular, I have been grateful for writings of Sam Keen, an American author, professor and philosopher. Keen is best known for his exploration of questions regarding being a male in a modern society. I have set this book firmly within the framework of his inspiration. In particular, I have appreciated his concepts in relation to creating the Exemplar or Ideal Man.

I am also grateful for the assistance of insightful colleagues who have agreed to be readers, in particular author and journalist Adrian McGregor, counsellor, leadership and executive coach Gail Intas, urologist and men's health advocate Emeritus Professor 'Frank' Gardiner AM and Kay McGrath OAM, co-chair of the Domestic and Family Violence Prevention Council for the Queensland Government.

I acknowledge the editorial assistance I have received from my editor, Joanne Holliman who has guided me wisely on content and design. In particular, I also must acknowledge publisher and editor Charli Fels for the tremendous counsel concerning audience targeting, titling and marketing strategies.

I must also acknowledge Sid Harta Publications' editor Tony Berry for his detailed and very professional final editing.

A special accolade also goes to my dedicated and ever-patient executive assistant Carol Marchant, whose experience in compiling the many drafts of this manuscript has been invaluable.

Peter Dornan AM
2023

Contents

Introduction		1
One	*The Dominant Feather*	19
Two	*The Belligerent Feather*	35
Three	*The Uncommunicative Feather*	48
Four	*The Repugnant Feather –*	
	Domestic Violence	60
Five	*The Exemplar Feather*	
	– Be a Positive Role Model	65
Six	*The Creative Feather*	75
Seven	*The Denial Feather*	
	– the Ivory Tower of Manhood	81
Eight	*The Catastrophic Feather*	
	– Find the Power Within	91
Nine	*The Burgeoning Feather*	
	– The Awakening and the	
	Mid-Life Crisis	101
Ten	*The Grieving Feather*	112
Eleven	*The Manly Feather*	122

Twelve	*The Avant-Garde Feather*	142
Thirteen	*The Kingly Man Feather*	152
Fourteen	*The Odyssean Feather*	
	– Roadmap for an Odyssey	160
Fifteen	*The Futuristic Feather*	164
Sixteen	*The Beseeching Feather*	
	– Ask for Help	171
Seventeen	*The feather of the stout-hearted men*	
	– find a support group	177
Eighteen	*The Loving Feather – Relationships*	183
Nineteen	*The Wild Feather – Go Wild*	198
Twenty	*The Healthy Feather*	212
Twenty-One	*The Newly Adorned Dashing Peacock*	234
Twenty-Two	*The Ancient Feather*	238

INTRODUCTION

*'Life is a competition of prattling peacocks
enraptured in inane mating rituals.'*
— Christopher Nolan

'A peacock? Who, me, a peacock?' He casts an artful, pleased look from the corner of his eye, admiring his presumptuous pose. He preens in front of the mirror.

'Yes. You – a peacock.'

'Well, I have got some very marvellous feathers.'

'I agree – you have some beautiful ones. But some are very dowdy. I reckon it's time to look at refeathering a few of them.'

'Dowdy? Dowdy? Which ones?'

'For starters, that one there – the invincible one. That screams "nothing can hurt me". The one that refuses to ask for help.'

'Really?'

'Yes, then there's the very outmoded dominant one. The one that says you must always be in charge and never wrong

'Then there is that very drab one – the uncommunicative one. It has forgotten how to listen and share stories. It spends far too much time working, denying time to understand the needs of your partner

'And this one here – very shabby and past its use-by date – the belligerent one. It fixes things by aggression

'And finally, this little one here. It lacks EI.'

'EI?'

'Emotional intelligence.'

'Oh. Not too sure what that means. What about the pretty ones?'

'As I said, you have some very beautiful ones plenty of them – loyal, shows respect, self-reliant, tenacious, courageous and steps up to a challenge. But you need to add some vibrant new ones.'

'Hmmm. How do I do that?'

'First, we need to assist you to come down out of your ivory tower of manhood.'

'What's that?'

And when you have reached the mountain top, then you shall begin to climb. – Kahlil Gibran.

*

From the security and comfort of my seat on the international flight to Nairobi, my attention was suddenly diverted and transfixed on the compelling vision materialising outside my window. The ancient snow-covered cone of Mt Kilimanjaro appeared and sparkled as it soared out of the Tanzanian plains below like a massive beacon. I felt I could almost stroke the snow as the captain obligingly banked and circled the plane above the rim of the crater to give us a better view.

Nudging 20,000 feet (6000 metres), the African continent's highest peak was impressively emerging below the level of our plane's flight path. I immediately felt pangs of excitement and some unease as I realised this was why I was here. In a few days, I would be scrambling over the same massive mountain and those same frigid-looking heights.

As the mesmerising sight faded from my vision, I lapsed into moments of reflection. Why was I here? The date was February 2003. I was a sports and exercise physiotherapist, about to turn sixty and approaching retirement age.

Critically, I was recovering from a prostate cancer diagnosis. The results of invasive radical surgical treatment left me struggling with serious side effects, including reactive depression. This had gravely impacted on my lifestyle, as well as my professional career, emotional health, exercise activity and sex life. I was shocked. As a health professional (and an anatomist), at the time of my diagnosis I knew nothing of my prostate, where it was or what it did. Worse, there was very little official information or support available to assist me.

Cancer had stripped me of my sense of control, essential to effective care; the question of how to restore it was seriously perplexing. As a male I lived the role of being averse to sympathy, wary of pity and in denial so that I knew almost nothing about cancer management.

Why was this? Why didn't I know these things? Why did men not know these things? Or talk about them? Being bothered by these persistent questions, I determined to be a force for change.

The road to recovery involved starting one of the first support groups for men (and their partners) diagnosed with prostate cancer in Australia. Our first aim was to educate ourselves and learn how to treat and manage the side effects. We then set out to create community awareness of all aspects of prostate cancer and to stimulate research into men's health concerns.

As tough as it seems, illness can provide us with the capacity to gain new insights and wisdom, to cut through the nonsense and sham. There is no one answer to allow us to achieve this. Everybody will have different strategies to cope with their losses. Basically, cancer enables us to think about what is important and to prioritise things, and people, in our life.

Seven years after my diagnosis and treatment, I now felt the need for a sense of closure, to celebrate my new life. I was nimble again, had vanquished my side effects and had developed purpose. I would climb Mt Kilimanjaro as a resolution and a satisfying challenge.

Why climb a mountain to prove anything? There is a 1923 often quoted line by George Mallory, an Everest mountaineer, 'Because it is there.'

Most people would consider the exercise to be irrational. There is an almost existential absurdity to it all. A rational person goes around a mountain.

Perhaps on one level, I saw some symbolism suggestive of the uphill climb cancer survivors must face and overcome. On another level, it was a chance to measure myself, to balance the depressing threat of my life from cancer with an elation for living.

I had also come to understand that a man's reach should exceed his grasp; it is imperative to keep striving, to keep fuelling the drive to survive, to struggle, to do better, to create and be fulfilled. Or as philosopher Sam Keen reminds us, search for the fire burning in our bellies. I needed to keep challenging myself – physically as much as intellectually.

Mt Kilimanjaro lies close to the equator, yet snow, ice and glaciers are found on its highest slopes. It provides incredible views of hundreds of square kilometres of surrounding countryside – thousands of metres below – as well as of surrounding mountain peaks, valleys and glaciers.

The sixty-kilometre climb to the summit takes you through a number of distinctly different climatic and vegetation zones. From beautiful rainforest, which is often hot and stifling, to windy moorland, alpine desert and, finally glaciers, ice and snow, where the temperature can drop as low as minus 20 deg Celsius.

At Nairobi, where my plane landed, I liaised with my local mountain guide and met the other two members of our team who happened to come from Brisbane, my home town. Julian was a very fit twenty-three-year-old international surfing champion, who coincidentally had attended my old school, Brisbane Boys' College. The other was his father, Peter. We bonded very quickly.

We travelled to our base at Moshi, a small village and the gateway to Kilimanjaro. The next morning, we awoke to the vision of Kilimanjaro towering over us, its cone lost in mists and clouds. In great spirits, we began our climb.

After four days of hard climbing and trekking, my adventure almost finished at our final camp at 4,545 metres. Feeling the need to relieve myself, I left our tent and wandered over to a precipice. At the edge, I was momentarily struck by the magnificent panorama thousands of feet directly below and beyond. I rested my climbing poles on a rough tuft of grass, then watched in horror as one of them slid off and tumbled into space.

Luckily, the pole caught in the only piece of shrubbery on the rock face, some two metres below me. Without the pole, I could not possibly continue climbing and it would be very difficult to negotiate the downward track without it.

At this altitude, there was only sparse vegetation, but I noticed an ancient gnarled tree with one branch curled down over the cliff face. I tested it with my left hand and it seemed to take my weight. Gripping the other pole in my right hand, I levered myself warily over the edge of the precipice, extremely mindful of the consequences if the branch cracked. I stretched until the point of the pole caught under the leather loop of the handle of its fallen partner, deliberately not focussing on the dizzying depths behind it.

I slowly manoeuvred the right-hand pole to waist height, precariously dangling the second one from it, then, with a strong wrist flick catapulted it up over my head. It did a brisk complete somersault and luckily landed right behind me. Gratefully, situation saved.

I then returned to our camp, where we were instructed to catch four hours' sleep.

Our guide would wake us at 10.30 pm, allow us a cup of tea, then lead us in darkness on a seven-hour trek directly to the summit in time for sunrise. We would then return to camp and have a break before continuing downhill on a five-hour walk to our next camp, below the height where we would be most likely to develop serious altitude sickness – a total of fifteen hours walking for the day.

We always knew this day would be hard and there were some anxious moments as we tried to sleep. We were all well aware that this is the stage when most deaths occur, and eighty per cent of climbers are forced down before reaching the summit. Sleep was difficult as these thoughts weighed heavily on my mind. In particular, it concerned me that, should altitude sickness become so severe as to cause cerebral or pulmonary oedema, skilled medical help was a least two days of swift hiking from here.

Snow had rolled in off the summit during the short night and the temperature had dropped to freezing. Wind snapped at our tents, whipping and cracking them and our anxiety increased. But joyously, when we were woken at 10.30 pm for our cup of tea, we were greeted by a beautiful full moon and a landscape bathed in white, interspersed with black rock.

As we climbed, the scene took on an eerie, almost surreal atmosphere. Down on the African plain, lights from the local villages twinkled back at us, as in a fairyland. To our left and below us, a violent thunderstorm built up, crashing its loud warning as lightning flashed and darted around the sky. It was quite magical.

By 3 am the moon had slipped behind the mountain and the scene suddenly turned chillingly dark. We switched on our head torches and continued trudging uphill, fighting against snow, rock, mud and very unstable scree. Breathing became difficult and every footstep was a major task. At our last camp I needed one or two breaths for each step. Now, close to the summit, I needed five breaths to sustain just one footstep.

At this stage, around the cone of the ancient volcano, an unspoken drama played out as at least a dozen international teams converged. Trails of light dotted the steep gradient as climbers desperately searching for oxygen and energy called on their every resource to commit to the summit. Sadly, some lights were seen to turn back, the effort too great. Julian's father, Peter, turned back here, sick with diarrhoea.

I now needed seven lungfuls of air for each step but, though exhausted, I still felt in control and knew I had some energy in reserve. I was grateful for our guide's continual reminder to climb: 'Polo, polo, polo', – slowly, slowly, slowly. Let your body adapt, a mantra I still refer to today during times of pressure. Finally, I reached the top at about 6.30 am, accompanied by an unsurpassed sense of relief and achievement.

Julian and I spontaneously implemented a timeless ritual. We performed the Brisbane Boys' College war cry. It simply seemed appropriate.

The date was the 14 February, St Valentine's Day. I was mindful of the love and support I had gleaned from my wife to achieve this moment; I walked quietly off into the snow and stood on the edge of the crater and tried to sing a love song. No words came out. I was overwhelmed with emotion and exhaustion. Warm tears melted the ice on my cheeks.

What a tremendous way to see Africa – from its roof. From its highest point, peering out into the mists of distance, and indeed time. It was not hard to imagine the teeming animals on the plains far below waking as the first rays of the sun ignited the ancient landscape. After all, this is where our species' life on earth began. The song *Morning has broken* must have been inspired by such an emotion '...like the first morning.'

At that stage, some seven years after treatment, I considered my triumph to be fairly complete.

My thoughts went back to a passage I was reminded of during my darkest hours. Friend, colleague and fellow cancer survivor ethicist Noel Preston, suggested I keep looking for "the gift in all this." He related that the writer John O'Donohue had once stated, 'Often the most wonderful gifts arrive in shabby packaging.' From the comfort of that moment and the state of my present good health, nothing I say should camouflage how shabby that packaging was. However, over time, the gifts have revealed themselves.

As I moved from loss to life, from woundedness to wholeness, and from longing to acceptance, Noel revealed another O'Donohue insight, 'As the body ages, the soul gains in richness, becoming deeper and stronger.' But the greatest gift to me was the renewed awareness that my need for family and friends was far greater than any other drive, need or ambition.

To consolidate my sense of closure, I granted my climbing boots to my helpful guide, who was grateful for them. I wouldn't be doing any more climbing.

I was quite wrong. The quote at the beginning of this chapter, by Kahlil Gilbran, is a metaphor which refers mainly to conquering a major challenge or adversity. Gilbran was a Lebanese-American who lived in the early twentieth century when not many people climbed real mountains. It implies that once you have reached the summit (of any challenge), that will not be enough.

You will need to navel gaze like an ascetic, or guru, and contemplate your new existence. This includes examining the layers of veneer that have been stripped away, allowing the creation of a new compass that will guide you in the future. To quote TS Eliot from *Little Gidding*,

> We shall not cease from exploration
> And the end of all our exploring
> Will be to arrive where we started
> And know the place for the first time.

On my return to Brisbane, as if experiencing a type of epiphany, I recommitted myself to expanding my influence and advocacy in matters concerning men's health and manhood. I needed to open pathways for men to understand more of what it means to be a male and to discriminate between what is real and what may be a social construct of who we are. Perhaps we may need to seriously examine our behaviour and then make recommendations concerning change.

My college friend Julian also appeared to experience a moment of enlightenment on his return from Kilimanjaro. He studied medicine at the University of Queensland, now specialises in emergency medicine and is happily married to an anaesthetist.

To explain a little more concerning male behaviour I will now introduce a couple of archetypical characters as they enact a sometimes-familiar scenario.

Emily braced in her car seat. She heard the screeching of brakes, felt the crashing thud and then listened to the tinkling of broken glass. Her husband Christopher had also heard the imminent roaring of the reversing car, then saw it racing towards their car. He braced as the impact threw him forward in his seat.

They witnessed the driver, Joshua, stagger out of his car. He was filthy angry, furrowed brow, his shoulders hunched and forearms tight as he clenched his fists.

Chris was having none of it. He searched for a spanner which he kept under his seat for such occasions, then jumped out of the car to confront the other man. His adrenaline was pumping and he didn't realise he was limping, having smashed his knee on the dashboard.

As they moved towards each other, Joshua stopped, lowered his hands and shook his head from side to side. Emily, horrified, heard him grunt something unintelligible. Chris also stopped, moved his spanner across to his left hand, grinned and extended his right hand. Emily also heard him grunt something.

Both men examined the damage, then hopped back into their cars. They then drove off, honour apparently settled.

Emily asked 'What happened?'

'After the initial shock the other guy realised it was his fault. He apologised and asked if I was okay, and could he help with the repairs,' Chris replied.

'He said all that?' she asked, incredulously.

'Well, not quite, but I knew what he meant.'

'What did you say?'

'I said, "it's only a flesh wound, no drama, and I can repair the light myself, easy".'

'Did you actually say that? I only heard a grunt.'

'Well, he knew what I meant.'

Two weeks later, Chris was still limping, in denial that his knee was a problem. When Emily prompted him to see a doctor, he testily said no. He would be okay, it was only a flesh wound.

Another two weeks passed, his pain and disability developed further and he was now short-tempered, tired from limping, which was now putting pressure on other joints and muscles. As a tradesman, he could not work. Emily again suggested he should get it treated.

'I'll be okay. It'll get better,' Chris said angrily. A habitual drinker, he started drinking more heavily to ease the pain and anxiety, waiting for things to improve.

By another two weeks, reactive depression was setting in. He was becoming extremely uncommunicative, quick to yell and slammed doors in response to any discussion. The weeks passed and when Emily again asked him about seeing a doctor he lashed out, hitting her on the shoulder. Filled with remorse and not being adequately equipped emotionally to handle the situation, he went back to his drinking.

Even considering the joshing licence I have taken, concerning men's minimal but efficient ability to communicate with each other, variations of this hypothetical scene are probably acted out regularly by males. The question is, why don't men look after their health better? Why do they not admit something is wrong? Why do they bury their heads in the sand when it comes to managing their physical and mental health?

Why do they not share emotions, or show weakness of any sort? Why do they need to feel invincible and not ask for help?

These questions are relevant even for younger men. More than forty per cent of men aged over forty suffer serious health problems, including heart disease, stroke and cancer.

Equally important, why do they think it is okay to violate their partner? Forty per cent of Australian women report violence over their lifetime, by physical or sexual harassment, discrimination, emotional, coercive or psychological abuse used in order to exercise men's power and control.

According to White Ribbon, a global social movement working to stop men's violence against women, twenty-five women in Australia have been killed in the first four months of this year (2024), allegedly at the hands of partners or exes. That is one woman every four and a half days.

Tired masculine traits like stoicism, independence and self-reliance can get in the way of seeking some of the answers. I contend many of the answers to these situations can be found in our ancestry. I argue that we may need to search back 200,000 years or more, to East Africa, when our direct ancestors, early

Homo sapiens, began to emerge as the dominant species on earth.

We have to discover what events ignited this resistant, patronising and potentially dangerous behaviour and, in the process, reveal why it has persisted right up to the present. For solutions, as the first chapter will reveal, we may have to draw an even longer bow, go back about two million years to when our ancestors began to stand erect.

The survival needs of these pre-history societies dictated that stronger, testosterone-endowed males, the hunters, assumed three main roles: the three Ps – to procreate, to protect and to provide. This helped their self-belief that they were invincible and the dominant ones in society. The role of the women of the tribe emerged to raise the children, look after the cave, gather plant-derived food and small animals, and look after everyone's health, including the males. I suggest in modern times that these male responsibilities (the three Ps) impoverish and alienate men.

I suspect we have now revealed two serious legacies. First, males have been held captive in an ivory tower of manhood, isolated from emotion, not allowed to cry or ask for help. If we show any signs of weakness, our tower, our castle and all that is in it, may be viewed as vulnerable.

Secondly, women have been perceived to be inferior, leading in many cultures to male dominance and a sober misperception of inequality. Women's subjugation was quite possibly a legacy of the physical nature of life in an era when such skills were a necessity for survival.

I have written this book to help others to connect with their own perceptions and to spark the change to these perceptions, and through this process, change male behaviour. In particular, to change male thinking and, sequentially, provoke a broader change in society's thoughts, actions, emotions and behaviours. I hope the concepts discussed may be useful for any male who may be conducive to refocussing their awareness of who they are. I am particularly concerned for men middle-aged and beyond. This is the demographic I consider to be most at risk of physical and mental health difficulties.

I also want to explore themes relating to male health. Men are more prone to heart attacks, diabetes, high blood pressure, are more likely to die of melanoma, and usually live four years less than women.

Around twenty-one per cent of males will develop cancer in their lifetime, and thirteen per cent will die from the disease. By comparison, around eighteen per cent of females will be diagnosed and nine per cent will die. The latest Australian Bureau of Statistics figures show a baby boy can expect to live to 81.3 years old, while a baby girl can expect to reach 85.4. Queensland Health suspects this is mainly because men fail to seek medical advice.

Suicide is the biggest killer of Australians aged fifteen to twenty-four, with males making up seventy-five per cent of all deaths. Data published by the Australian Bureau of Statistics has shown men over eighty-five years of age have suicide rates more than three times the average. The silent challenge for men aged over eighty-five who take their own lives is psychological and existential distress, which can reinforce feelings of loneliness and worthlessness. As researcher Adrienne Withall notes, older men at risk of suicide may feel they are "no longer needed" or perceive themselves as "burdensome" to family and community.

These beliefs can overlap with major life transitions, such as retirement, stopping driving or moving to residential care, where they are a minority. Such stressful events can increase feelings and marginalisation, loss of independence and worthlessness.

A large scale longitudinal research on risks of suicide among cancer patients in the United States found that of 8.6 million patients, studied over nearly forty years, more than 13,000 died from suicide and eighty-three per cent were men.

Simply, we do not look after ourselves well enough – our "we'll be right" syndrome, male denial or more realistically, maybe our unawareness, has to be challenged.

In the following chapters, I discuss effects of a hypokinetic lifestyle, including obesity and its sequelae, mental health considerations focussing on depression and suicide and management of prostate cancer and erectile dysfunction. I also discuss the search for a balanced and dynamic lifestyle. This includes understanding male behaviour. I examine relationships, particularly discussing domestic violence.

Males initially need to understand what it is to be a male. To appreciate "manhood", we have to shed layers of stereotypes including myths of who we are and particularly discard our macho mantle. Machoism presents as an assertive exaggerated masculinity; men who swagger in an aggressive dominating manner, alpha males unaware of their potential vulnerability, men who suppress emotion. Toxic machoism emphasises the harmful effects of conforming to these ideals, along with related traits such as misogyny and homophobia, due in part to the promotion of violence including sexual assault and domestic violence.

Aggression is not a male trait, or vulnerability a female trait. These are not gender roles, but human qualities. Male vulnerability did not disappear, it just became naturally suppressed, thus rendering us emotionally powerless when we are confronted with any threatening situation or disease.

In this context, I suspect we will need to nurture and grow our emotional intelligence. Emotional intelligence is the capability of individuals to recognise their own emotions and those of others, discern between different feelings and label them appropriately using the emotional information to guide thinking and behaviour. To do this, we need to seek knowledge and apply it with experience and judgment, an entity which can only be effective coming from a solid base of values. Neuroscience posits that consequential thinking doesn't happen for males until around the age of twenty-seven. Small wonder they take actions which they may later regret, such as risk taking on the road, diving into pools without looking, shooting or punching first etc.

These assertions do not imply that the majority of males are not aware of the situation, or even that they are unhappy with their lot. Indeed, as one anonymous observer has commented, with some tongue in cheek levity (and I suspect the writer was a female), there are many reasons men as a whole present as happy people. The writer contends that this is what we should expect, from such simple creatures:

- The garage is all yours.
- Wedding plans take care of themselves.
- Chocolate is just another snack.
- Car mechanics tell you the truth.
- The world is your urinal.
- You never have to drive to another gas station restroom because this one is too icky.

- You don't have to stop and think which way to turn a nut on a bolt.
- Wedding dress – $5000. Tux rental – $100.
- People never stare at your chest when you're talking to them.
- Phone conversations are over in thirty seconds flat.
- A five-day vacation requires only one suitcase.
- You get extra credit for the slightest act of thoughtfulness.
- Your underwear is $8.95 for a three pack.
- Two pairs of shoes are more than enough.
- You are unable to see wrinkles in your clothes.
- The same hairstyle lasts for years, maybe decades.
- You can play with toys all your life.
- You can do Christmas shopping for twenty-five relatives on December 24 in twenty-five minutes.
- A man will pay $2 for a $1 item he needs. A woman will pay $1 for a $2 item that she doesn't need, because it is on sale.
- A man has six items in his bathroom; a toothbrush and toothpaste, a razor, soap, deodorant and a towel. The average number of items in a typical woman's bathroom is 337. A man would not be able to identify more than twenty of these items.
- A woman will dress up to go shopping, water the plants, empty the trash, answer the phone, read a book and get the mail. A man will dress up for weddings and funerals.

To fulfil these aspirations we have first to look beyond the fables. We need to ask serious questions, such as what is a male? What is masculinity? What role does this play with aggression and with our tendency to be in denial in matters relating to our health and our relationships with women?

So allow me to present my insights about the notion of all things manhood, from ancient to modern.

Let me start by finding out who we are. Let me present, an historical perspective on the journey of manhood. Hopefully this may enlighten where we have come from, understanding our past to inform the future.

During our expedition, I will explore such issues as identity, relationships, general health, male medical conditions and mental health mindset, depression, suicide etc as well as sexual activity and erectile dysfunction.

From here, I would like to assume a turning point. It has been suggested males, like peacocks, may attempt to mesmerise by brilliantly displaying colourful, flashy feathers. As such, some cultures consider the peacock to be associated with benevolence, patience, kindness and compassion. These are surely desirable feathers. However, it has also been suggested some of these flashy feathers, and some not so flashy, have become dowdy and well past their use by date. It is time to advocate some beautiful new modern ones.

So let's consider we are on the cusp, a transitioning. Let's continue the journey by proposing a future where we have control to reject, redefine and reimage a modern male.

CHAPTER ONE

The Dominant Feather

Where have we come from? *Homo sapiens*: wise man.

It is a well-used template: 'He struts on to the stage, proud as a peacock.' This simile alludes to the male peacock with its elaborate wooing rituals, its swaggering stance and its colourful tail, the exhibition vividly displaying his impressive, iridescent feathers adorned with brilliant eyespots. This posture and pageantry have long symbolised vanity, pride, dominance and excessive self-esteem.

Where did this idea of male dominance come from?

I suspect a good place to start would be in pre-history. We should visit East Africa, the Savannah, 200,000 years ago, the era of our ancestors, the hunter-gatherers.

This is a period when groups of males, the hunters, would venture into the wilds to secure a large animal as a meal for the tribe. These men, the hunters, had become endowed with increased testosterone enabling them to become taller, stronger and invariably, risk-takers.

The hunter-gatherers' language was adequate to set basic mythic rules of hierarchy and agree to concepts of law and leadership – and to establish the pecking order. It also allowed them to describe and accept social roles for survival, including gender status, and the responsibility of elders. Everyone had a role to enable sustainability that was rarely challenged. Even though there was a fair amount of personal independence, there was no such concept of individual rights. The system had evolved from the historical necessity of protecting the tribe, the font of their existence.

Let me articulate some speculative observations.

I suspect this was an important era for certain roles and behaviours to be conditioned into the system. I consider this may be the defining era where men distinctly merged into their perceived role of the three Ps – to procreate, protect and provide.

Let us go back much further. When elements of our life, yours, mine and all other life forms on earth began 3.8 billion years ago, we reproduced by asexual reproduction (simple cell division). This method was used until two billion years ago when the first eukaryotes (organisms whose cells have a nucleus) engaged in sex, as our common ancestors found we could evolve faster by sexual reproduction. For the ancestors of our specific species, up until about two million years ago, we could speculate males and females were generally equal, dancing around each other, moving in and out of polygamous and monogamous relationships.

We can also speculate males and females both participated in subsistence gathering for their communities during this period. As the environment changed, and we adapted, random mutations created a situation where our gender roles were dramatically transformed.

I suspect these tendencies would have been accelerated when our ancestors first stood up, *Homo erectus*, two million years ago. This ability changed many things including the nature of birth, as will be seen further on, and the dynamics of the tribe.

These three roles, procreate, protect and provide, are what

males needed to be good at. For survival and for our species to emerge dominant, variations of this structure, including inequities, continued with little change down through the centuries. This system worked like a giant anthill, or beehive, in which everybody had their role and function, pledged for the higher interests of the tribe. Individuality was not encouraged.

We have lived by these three Ps through the generations. Males continued to identify with the three Ps even with the emergence of the cognitive revolution about 70,000 years ago, an era when our brains amazingly developed massive improvements to our cognitive abilities and allowed our achievements to set us up definitively as the dominant species

We resolutely followed this concept from the savannas and jungles of Africa, during the frozen ice ages of Europe, from hunting mammoths through to hunting buffalo on the American plains, to fishermen at sea, to modern corporate warriors circling a good deal or, to take a rather large leap, engaging in the ultimate gladiator sport of politics.

This cemented in the tribal consciousness, a situation whereby men assumed a perceived dominant role as an extension of their vital protective behaviour. Women, on the other hand, accepted a more reproductive, nurturing, vulnerable and subservient role in most, but not all circumstances; a perceived inferior position which necessitated the need to be provided for and protected.

In nearly all other mammals, the offspring are raised by the mother alone. The male is generally only useful as a sperm bank, a situation where he competes, often aggressively, and often to the death, to be top of the gene pool.

In the hunter-gatherer *Homo sapien*s state, a single mother could not provide enough high quality food or protection for her infants from other males. This is a trade-off for our specie's ability to stand erect. During this process our pelvic bones narrowed and babies were born prematurely; they could not exit the pelvis easily and so needed to arrive early. This meant they had to be looked after for some time after birth. In contrast, many mammals have longer gestation periods compared with humans. Examples of this include gorillas, elephants, sperm whales, walruses, giraffes, camels and zebras.

These events also set in motion the woman's role. They looked after and raised the children, organised the orderly running of the settlement (or cave) and were the gatherers of local food, nuts, berries and fruit. They also morphed into the role of looking after the health of everyone, including the men. This was probably an obvious role. They knew the medicinal herbs, flowers, opiates and anti-inflammatories etc. They witnessed and observed firsthand sickness and could predict prognostic clinical pathways. While the men were out hunting all day, the women developed empathic, nurturing and caring ways. In the same way, the males would have developed strong mateship values.

Because of this multi-skilling I would also suggest women probably developed wider social skills, female intuition and guile and a more expansive language base than men. There is recent evidence which, to a certain extent, challenges the hypothesis of man-the-hunter model. The research, along with other articles, some published in *Science Advances*, reports the discovery of a female body buried in the Americas some 9,000 years ago alongside hunting tools. The authors propose this may mean big game hunting was indeed carried out by men and women in hunter gatherer groups.

It is tempting to suggest that what happened in the paleolithic era is up for grabs. However, this concept is supported by further recent research by University of Delaware anthropology professor Sarah Lacy and her colleague Cara Ocobock from the University of Notre Dame (Phys.org. 20 October 2023). Through a review of current archaeological evidence and literature, they found little evidence to support the idea that roles were assigned specifically to each sex. They proffer that in a small society everyone has to be able to pick up any role at any time.

Regardless, I suspect the notion that males may have acquired the impression they were ascendant had less to do with the fact that they may, or may not, have been hunters. I suspect it was more that they were simply bigger and stronger and assumed the role of protectors and therefore were "in charge".

Subsequently the establishment of agriculture and abandonment of nomadic, hunter-gathering practices resulted in permanent settlements.

These led to a need for different attributes in physical and mental behaviour. Protection of people and property fell exclusively to males. For an effective army, a chain of command was essential with regimentation of fighting troops. Soldiers included commandeered peasants, serfs, slaves and others under the direction of a controlling elite. Women continued to provide a supporting role in many ways, much as they continue to do today, although a minority now fulfill more active "warrior" roles along with men.

The status of women varied across the ancient world. For example, in ancient Egypt women could acquire wealth. They could buy and sell property, slaves, servants and livestock and a woman could inherit part of her husband's estate. Furthermore, women could play an active role in legal proceedings. In ancient Mesopotamia, most women were subjugated by denial of a lack of autonomy. A woman was regarded as a father's daughter or a husband's wife. However, a number of those in the powerful and ruling elite had greater privileges such as being able to inherit a husband's estate in the absence of male heirs. Nevertheless, their rights and privileges were considerably less than those of men of similar social standing.

While the past, as quoted by British novelist, LP Hartley is a foreign country, community-wide participation makes good evolutionary sense. However, even though this may have been a possibility in that era, in most modern societies, women were shielded from heavy tasks, athletic endeavour and risky activities. For instance, women were not allowed to compete at the ancient Olympic Games, traditionally dated to 776 BC, through to AD 394, more than a thousand years ago.

When the modern Olympic Games began in 1896, 245 athletes came from fourteen different countries – but no women. Misogyny was entrenched.

Women were admitted in 1900 in sports that were considered compatible with their femininity and fragility, but were excluded from the showpiece events of track and field. In 1960, women were allowed to compete in the 800 metres. It wasn't until 2007, that the Olympic charter made the presence of women mandatory in every sport.

Even in my era, growing up in the 1950s, when I attended a one-teacher school in Western Queensland, on our one sports day of the year, boys (up to Grade 8, fourteen years) could compete in the sprint (80 yards) and the high jump and broad jump. Girls could only do a fifty-yard sprint, tunnel ball and potato races, but no jumps. It was considered unladylike and the impact may injure their pelvis.

Since early pre-historic days, it has generally been men who have made the laws, set the agendas and, with few exceptions, most societies have been patriarchal. Even Aristotle (384-322 BC), one of the greatest rational thinkers, scientists and philosophers of all time, the originator of the study of logic, believed in the natural inferiority of women, reflecting the prevailing view of his time.

Patriarchy endures. The most common injustice seen around the world is the exclusion of women from humanity's ledger of rewards and opportunities.

Men owned the land, goods, chattels and women. Until the beginning of the 20th century, women (half the population) could not vote. Any goods they had belonged to their husband and they rarely could borrow money, implying it was difficult ever to acquire wealth. They were denied equal access to the right to vote and to political powers, and still are in some cultures. They were made to work harder and compensated less. Their best chance in life was to marry well.

This vision and situation has persisted until recently in most developed countries and, increasingly, in others. For most of recorded history women have been seen as subjugated by men. However, during the 18th century, the justice of this arrangement began to be openly challenged. Among the most prominent voices of dissent was that of the English radical Mary Wollstonecraft. I do like her famous quote from 1792, 'The mind will ever be unstable that has only prejudice to rest on.'

Many previous thinkers had cited the physical differences between the sexes to justify the social inequality between women and men. However, in the light of new ideas that had been formulated during the 17th century, such as John Locke's view that nearly all knowledge was acquired through experience and education, the validity of such reasoning was put into question.

Wollstonecraft argued that if men and women are given the same education, they will acquire the same good character and rational approach to life because they have fundamentally similar brains and minds. She demanded that women be treated as equal citizens with men, with equal legal, social and political rights. Her protestations sowed the seeds of the suffragette and feminist movements that were to flourish in the 19th and 20th centuries. In essence, the sentiment promoted is the right of women to control their own bodies, minds and lives.

This momentum really started towards the end of the 19th century when women in several countries had won the right to vote. The very first time that it was specifically written into a constitution that all men and all adult women (over eighteen years and all indigenous) were enfranchised to vote for the head of their ruling executive was Pitcairn, in 1838. Fifty-one years earlier this tiny island in the South Pacific was the refuge for nine mutineers from *HMS Bounty*. (Linda Colley, *The Gun, the Ship and the Pen*).

After Pitcairn, New Zealand in 1893 was the first country in the world to allow women to vote. The colony of South Australia followed in 1894. After federation in Australia, in 1901, women (only white ones, I might add) had the right to vote. But it took until 1962 for indigenous women to establish this right.

This impetus and energy continued with Emmeline Pankhurst

in the late 19th century, leading the fight for women's suffrage in England, a war that began with women heckling politicians and chaining themselves to railings. The resistance graduated to burning down buildings and blowing up empty churches in the middle of the night. Pankhurst finally forced her government in 1918 to give the vote to women who had reached thirty years of age. The writer, Grantlee Kieza, noted that Pankhurst, regarded by opponents in her lifetime as a dangerous ratbag, is now widely revered as one of the most influential women of the 20th century.

The push for women's suffrage in the United States began in 1848. Two socially active women, Elizabeth Cady Stanton and Lucretia Mott, indignant at the limitations of what women were able to achieve, organised America's first convention on women's rights.

The women drafted a 'Declaration of Sentiments' to be presented to the convention for approval. Modelled on the US Declaration of Independence, the document decried men's "absolute tyranny" over women, citing grievances that reflected the very limited rights women in America had at that time As noted by Rachel Hartigan in her essay "The Fight To Be Heard", published in the August 2020 edition of the *National Geographic*, married women were "civilly dead" because they did not have legal rights separate from their husband. Nor could they own property or even keep the wages they'd earned themselves. Colleges were closed to women; so were professions. 'Man,' the declaration stated, 'has endeavoured in every way that he could, to destroy (women's) confidence in her own power, to lessen her self-respect and to make her willing to lead a dependant and abject life.'

It took more than seventy years, until 1920 for (white) women in the United States to finally gain access to the ballot. This was in the wake of the devastation of the First World War and the Spanish Flu pandemic of 1918. The two crises opened the American labour market to women and exposed gender inequities that would no longer stand when the war ended and influenza abated. For the rest of the women in minority groups – black women, Chinese Americans and Native Americans, – it took until Congress's passage of the Voting Rights Act of 1965 for them finally to be able to vote.

One of the most important radical changes occurred in 1975 when Ruth Bader Ginsburg forced changes to the constitution regarding discrimination on the basis of sex (gender).

There are many other extraordinary women who gave birth to the feminist movement. Emma Miller, Simone de Beauvoir Adrienne Rich, Vida Goldstein, Annie Lowe, Frances Harper, Ida B Wells etc. They have added the words "free", "equal" and "powerful" to the definition of "woman" for all time.

With the advent and success of the suffragettes, what is known now as the Third Wave of the Feminist Movement, the Pill (contraception), MeToo Movement, and with the force of many other Women's organisations, gender equality has gained much traction. Attitudes to marriage, living together, sexuality, amongst other issues, have altered greatly over recent decades. These changes, along with most people now living in urban societies, mean demands on men for providing and protecting are not as great as previously in history.

There is still a large difference in corporate, political and leadership roles, wages and many other facets, including sport, yet this is slowly changing. Women, and men, are working with government and business to move from incremental gains to a systemic change and thus build a future in which women and men have equal social and economic choices and responsibilities. Although change is predicted to be slow, the increasing number of nations with female leaders such as Thatcher, May and Truss in the UK, Gandhi (India), Meir (Israel), Gillard (Australia), Arden (NZ) and Harris (USA) to name but a few, indicates the pace of change may be quickening.

The World Economic Forum states that gender parity in our lifetime is unlikely. In fact, the Global Gender Gap Report 2020 reveals that gender parity will not be attained for 99.5 years. Further, the Georgetown Institute for Women, Peace and Security reported that for 2019, women's representation in government was an average share of 21.5 per cent in national legislation worldwide.

The report predicts at the current pace it will take fifty-two years to reach gender parity. At present only two countries have more than fifty per cent. In Australia's Federal Parliament, the Senate hit gender parity for the first time in 2019, and thirty per cent of lower house MPs are women. It is of some local pride that my home state of Queensland in Australia has fifty per cent in our State Government and we have had two female premiers.

However, there are signs that Australian companies are making progress, at least at the board level. In 2020, women represented twenty-six per cent of recent board appointments in ASX 200 companies and thirteen per cent of total director positions, up from eight per cent in early 2010. What is interesting is that women and men do not have materially different levels of ambition. Seventy-four per cent of women and seventy-six per cent of men in a recent survey aspire to leadership roles. However, it is regularly stated that leadership should be based on merit, not gender, race and religion etc.

Even so, there is a wide gap between intention and outcome. In a 2011 global report by Bain & Company, two major issues appear to hold women back. First there is the perception about the challenges associated with competing work-life priorities, that is juggling work and family and choosing to prioritise a more balanced lifestyle. The other factor concerns differences in style as the critical inhibitor. Business men and women who answered a survey consider women undersell their experience and capabilities and some leadership teams do not value the different perspectives that women bring to the team. (And men often oversell – bluff!).

Another important fact limiting promotion is that men in senior roles are more likely to appoint or promote someone with a style similar to their own. Women don't typically fit the bill – they work differently, behave differently and are less comfortable promoting their ability.

Importantly, as the Bain & Company report notes, there is no gender difference in attributes such as making commercially sound decisions, but they achieve these outcomes with quite different styles. Simply put, women collaborate more whereas men promote their points of view more effectively. The report also noted men appear to be more effective at speaking up at a meeting and managing emotions at work.

It is also well documented that men talk over women (manterruptions – see below). Research shows in the workplace they talk eighty-one per cent more than women.

Language study expert Roly Sussex relates there are some new terms for men behaving inappropriately in conversations, although, the behaviours themselves are old.

One of these is manterrupting, when a man heedlessly and needlessly interrupts a woman. The man may have something to add, or not, but he interrupts anyway.

Then there is bropropriating, or taking over a woman's ideas after she presented them but been virtually ignored.

And now there is mansplaining, when a man takes it upon himself to explain something to a woman that the woman already knows and which may well be something that women would normally know more about than men.

Along these lines, researcher Sam Keen noted there was also the mistaken belief that women would change the rules of business and bring a moderate form of communication and human kindness into the boardroom. Keen notes this hasn't happened yet. Women executives have proved themselves to be the equal of men in every way, including callousness. He observes that the differences between the sexes are being eroded as both genders become defined by work. The corporate person, male or female, is in danger of becoming a being who has been neutralised, degendered and rendered subservient to the laws of the market. He suggests it has the potential to destroy the fullness of manhood and womanhood.

Regardless, in 2020, research from the Australian Government Workplace Gender Equality Agency, delivered a clear message: More women in key decision-making positions deliver better company performance, greater productivity and greater profitability.

The research analysed changes in the gender composition

of leadership structures within a company and linked these to company performance. It demonstrated that increasing the representation of women across key leadership roles added company market value of between $52 million and $70 million a year for an average sized organisation.

Further, the Chief Executive Women organisation reported further key findings from the above agency: having a female CEO of an Australian ASX-listed company led to a five per cent increase in company market value. This is worth the equivalent of $79.6 million on average.

On another level, women are making strides in space missions. NASA's plans for the Artemis Mission 3 involves the goal of landing 'the first woman and the next man' on the moon by 2025. This will be the first landing since Apollo 17 Mission in December 1972.

Everyone has a role to play in achieving gender equality. There are four priority areas which have recently been identified and targeted in the push for change.

- Participation and leadership – where women and girls participate fully and equally in society and leaders in the community, in politics and business.
- Economic security – society must work for women to achieve economic security across their life.
- Safety – women need to feel secure (in car parks, buses, parks) and have access to legal and justice services.
- Health and wellbeing – women should be encouraged to be healthy, well and active.

Change generally has also revved up for males as well, most accepting the changing roles and many celebrating the refreshing vision brought by females.

However, in some Eastern and Western, as well as some religious cultures, there is still strong resistance to such transformation.

At the deepest level, observers document that the gravest human rights issue in our country is domestic violence. Australia's former Governor-General Quentin Bryce said domestic violence was 'about men having power and control.' She continued, 'Among some men there's a backlash against the advancements and progress of women gaining power and leadership, and how their roles have changed. It's ownership, ... Women are possessions and the males own them. Men who abuse women have very grave issues of self-control, anger and power. There is a lot of anger around.'

The question is asked, 'Are men really so intolerant? Even lousy?'

If the answer is yes, why is this so?

First, let us examine what defines a male. Typically, and initially, the prime role for any male is that he has the capacity to produce spermatozoa, which fertilises the eggs of a female. Second, we have to look at what defines "manhood".

Manliness, masculinity and manhood are all reasonably interchangeable terms related to the state or period of being a man, rather than a child. Over generations, men have adapted to and generally exhibited a certain behaviour set in motion by our pre-history ancestors.

Twelve years ago, columnist Rory Gibson was given a brief: 'Give women an insight into how men think.' With some humour and tongue in check, he said he would set his writing around these pretexts.

1. All men are perves, but some hide it better than others.

2. You can ask us to do anything, just don't tell us how to do it.
3. Chick flicks: men secretly love them because they are like training manuals to help us understand women.
4. If a man is watching the footy, and it's five minutes from full time with the scores all locked up, that is not the time to start a conversation about getting new bath towels.
5. Throw pillows – WTF? (For male readers, "Throw" pillows are decorative pillows loosely tossed on sofa's, beds, floors).

It would appear men are so predictable concerning our behaviour patterns, Gibson is still writing along these themes with insight and humour, a tricky thing to do in this age of heightened sensibilities and people easily taking offence.

Let us look at some other feathers, but first, if you'd like to read an expanded story of the hunter-gatherers, I have included a bonus chapter at the end of the book – "The Ancient Feather".

CHAPTER TWO

The Belligerent Feather

'Strength does not have to be belligerent and loud,'
— **Russell Brand.**

It is well documented that peacocks may behave affectedly in a belligerent fashion.

My introduction to real belligerence began abruptly and unexpectedly as a thirteen-year-old boarder at high school. Until then I had attended a one-teacher country school and never having been intimidated or threatened.

In the first two weeks as a boarder, new students were expected to undergo initiation ceremonies, a bizarre tradition that I wasn't prepared for. It was a decades old culture inherited from military institutions that was designed to teach military-style discipline through a chain of command, a means to instil obedience.

This closed system generally involved degrading procedures operated by the senior boys, away from teachers. Generally, the new student was forcibly restrained and had their private parts painted with toothpaste or shoe polish. This was usually carried out in the locker room, often at shower time.

When it came my turn, I resisted strongly. Several boys grabbed me by the arms, locking them, and tried to force me to the ground. I was having none of it. I was able to thrust one boy backwards and at the same time freed my other hand. My ire up, I came out swinging wildly, an innate survival reaction I didn't know was there. Next thing, the boys released me and formed a ring, shouting, 'Fight, fight!'

This was new to me as I had never been in a fight. I suddenly felt a cold panic. There was nowhere to go. Primal fear now fuelled my will to protect myself. I threw punches from everywhere and within a few minutes, the boy was on the ground calling me to stop.

I didn't enjoy the experience, but I did learn about the benefit of assertion. I realised youthful male culture appreciated the "have a go" attitude; the incident immediately endowed me with some respect.

When I had calmed down, I wasn't too concerned by the event. I considered it was simply a rite of passage, a form of acceptance by my peers. However, deep down, I was quietly troubled as I was aware a lot of boys could be broken by this experience. I made up my mind never to inflict this on anybody else. (Some years later, the school did likewise and this tradition has been outlawed for many years).

However, I needed to be prepared next time. The school had a martial arts program where boys could learn the 'manly and noble art' of boxing, or judo, with the idea of being able to defend oneself.

I chose to learn boxing. I stayed with the boxing squad for the whole four years at school and enjoyed punching a bag and attaining the high level of discipline and fitness required. I became the school champion in my division every year, including welterweight in the final year.

I continued boxing when I left school and trained under one of Australia's top boxing trainers and promoters, Reg Layton. By the end of the year, I had developed in strength, speed, agility and skill and at eighteen I considered I was ready for the state boxing titles. Reg thought otherwise. He said I was, 'Too green and not ready.' He asked his other trainer, Johnny Green, to be my second in the ring.

However, in my own mind, I was ready. In the final, I was to meet the undefeated Queensland Golden Gloves Champion, Bobby J. Bobby who, at the age of twenty-one was favoured to win and compete in the Commonwealth Games team for Perth the next year in 1962.

I didn't have proper boxing clothes or boots, only my town desert shoes and football shorts and was taken lightly by Bobby. I had brought my dad along and he was sitting a couple of rows from the front.

I was exceedingly nervous, to the point of nausea and had to relieve myself (defecate) three times shortly before entering the ring. From the opening bell, Bobby started to play with me, boxing to the letter, searching for an opening. Once again, I was having none of it. I raced at him furiously, punching hard and fast, hitting him in the face and the chest several times. He was shocked and completely overwhelmed. Within twenty seconds, he dropped to the floor.

He groggily stood up and took the count to eight, shook his head, then came back, determined to give me a lesson. Once again, I was having none of it. I smashed fiercely into any gap he had open, causing him for a second to drop his guard protecting his head. I lashed out with a strong right haymaker and knocked him clear under the ropes, out of the ring and on to the floor. The bout was over.

I was now the state welterweight boxing champion. I would now be in the team to fight in the nationals in Perth for a chance to represent Australia. But it wasn't as easy as that. Dad was proud on one hand but was concerned about the sport. The next day, he followed through and found Bobby had gone to hospital after the fight. He had serious concussion and I had broken his jaw in five places. He was never going to fight again and retired from boxing.

Mum and dad were not impressed. Dad said, 'Son, you've got a good brain, you should use it. You should retire.' I had strong regrets and struggled. However, I did respect my father's counsel. I did retire.

With sport, there is a degree of triumph, a feeling of elation, a victory to reach for and to push for the boundaries of performance, skills, strength, speed and endurance. There are going to be winners and losers, and injuries. But and with the coming of maturity I now fully understand that to dominate by exhibiting assertiveness and destroying the opponent's brain is nothing less than barbarism ,and is no better than an organised physical assault.

The Association of Neurological Surgeons states that nearly ninety per cent of boxers suffer a brain injury of some extent during their career (14 January 2013).

I still shadow box and punch, without actually hitting someone, but I do keep my body fit and responsive and, in an imperfect world, prepared for self-defence.

Research has clearly shown that every blow kills brain cells, and the aim of these sports is, primarily to paralyse, to knock opponents down or out. The rules have recently been changed around head hits in rugby league and other major football codes.

There is now a whole generation of footballers from the 1960s, many suffering dementia from the abuse caused by concussion. There is also emerging evidence that repetitive belts on the head by a ball has a deleterious effect on soccer players.

How did we develop this behaviour? This need to be always in control – to be top of the pecking order. Is our behaviour a result of the primitive brain overriding the cortical? Is it in our trace memory? Or is it irrevocably embedded in our DNA? Is it the result of millions of years of random mutations ensuring an advantage by being stronger and faster, becoming necessary risk-takers with a propensity for aggression and conflict? And the need to be in power? Or could it be that in an era when physical strength is not such an advantage, some men feel threatened, potentially rendering them dangerous?

Even to ask the question and expect a reasonable answer could be construed to resemble peacock thinking. I suspect this situation relates a little to the well-known "Starfish Story".

An old man, a writer, lived on a beach overlooking the ocean. He would walk along the beach every morning for inspiration. One morning, after a massive storm, he noticed the beach was littered with thousands of starfish. Up ahead, he noticed a boy pick up a starfish and throw it gently into the ocean. Approaching the boy, he asked, 'What are you doing'?

The youth replied, 'Throwing starfish back into the ocean. The surf is up and the tide is going out, if I don't throw them back, they'll die.'

'Son,' the man said, 'Don't you realise there are thousands of starfish on this beach? You can't make a difference.'

After listening politely, the boy bent down, picked up another starfish and threw it back into the surf. Then, smiling at the man, he said, 'I made a difference to that one.'

So we might have to make a difference – to one man at a time.

Researcher Chip Brown considers that anthropologists and sociologists generally tend to consider our behaviour derives more from culture. He suspects it is developed from learning, from being carefully taught, believing that masculinity is something constructed by cultures and must be earned and proved. Rigid fundamentalist religious cultures and dogma tend also to reinforce the attitude that men should be dominant.

'Men are made, not born,' argues Michael Kimmel, a professor of sociology at Stony Brook University, New York. 'Manhood is not a manifestation of an inner essence….it does not bubble up to consciousness from our biological constitution; it is created in our culture.'

Throughout history, cultures have devised myriad practices and rituals to make boys into men. The methods, often secret, sacred and painful, vary widely and share universal themes that broadly reflect a community's values and the roles men are expected to play, says anthropologist Gilbert Herdt.

This may be true. Since the days when we became aware of our overarching male responsibilities, we have been programmed to approach our existence through the lenses of warfare and work. In fact, the three Ps could be translated to three Ws – Women, Work and War.

War and fighting have always been part of the human experience. The 'P' of protection, which incorporated a degree of fighting, merged into 'W' for warfare over many generations. For hundreds of thousands of years the hunter-gatherers lived within the seasons of nature. As nomads, they were extremely conservative and were relatively harmonious with other tribes apart from an occasional fleeting conflict, and existed in realms confident that nature would supply enough. No need to innovate, simply do things the way they have always been done.

This concept of sacred respect for the land and its fauna and flora, still resonates with indigenous tribes today. As quoted by legendary Indian leader and powerful environmentalist Chief Seattle (1786-1866), 'The earth does not belong to man, man belongs to the earth. All things are connected, like the blood that unites us all. Man did not weave the web of life; he is merely a strand in it. Whatever he does to the web, he does to himself.'

However, about 12,000 years ago, in the Fertile Crescent region of the Middle East, this all changed. The hunter-gatherers began to harvest wild grains such as wheat and barley that they found growing there. They became agriculturists. They began to live in settled communities and grew crops or raised animals on nearby land. In Mesopotamia, 5000 years ago, these small tribes unified into the first urban centres of larger national communities with a rich, complex and varied life. They eventually grew into cities where lofty ziggurats, or temple towers, rose skyward, art and technological ingenuity blossomed, and individual specialisation and commercial enterprise changed the arena in which manhood was to develop.

The individual warrior, the protector, steadily became part of larger warfare units in which behaviour was regimented for an effectiveness mostly lost in hierarchical organisation. Political loyalty was no longer to the tribe or clan but to the wider community as a whole. This was also the period where, over some millennia, the connections to the sanctity of the earth were replaced by transcendent male gods who encouraged men to create their own destiny.

Our early hunter-gatherer ancestors would have gazed into the brilliant night sky, ablaze with a canopy of stars, constellations, galaxies, shooting stars and the moon and tried to reason their own existence in a bewildering cosmos. They clearly lived in an intimacy with nature in which every aspect of their life, the animals, trees, rocks, were connected to the earth. In this process, they developed a bond to the Earth Mother, the supplier of all their needs, the Earth Goddess. However, being mesmerised by the infinite mystery of this extra-terrestrial display surely would have prompted the concept that maybe superior overlords played and lived in the heavens, manifested through polytheism, and maybe had an influence on their lives.

In Mesopotamia's early cities, Sumaria and Babylon, the invention of a practical writing system allowed these now better educated men to record their thoughts. It was here that a celestial order was created to form a common vision to unite them. This way, they could place in authority systems to maintain laws, stores, grains, homes and people.

According to Sumerian legend, Enlil, the god of the air and storms, separated the heavens, the domain of his father, An, from the earth, which was the realm of his mother, the goddess Ki. An offered the promise of a heavenly existence as a reward for a tough life. This concept was not only the realm of the Sumerians.

In ancient Egypt, Amun-Ra, king of the gods, was the supreme creator god. He offered the same reward to kings. For the Vikings, Odin and his son Thor lived in the kingdom of Asgard in the sky. Odin's wife Frigg was more closely associated with the earth.

Warriors who died in battle were transported by Valkyries to Valhalla, a majestic hall in Asgard, to a Norse heaven. For the Greeks, Zeus was the reigning god. He sent dead Greek warriors to paradise, the fields of Elysian, to be conferred with immortality. And for the Romans, Jupiter, father of the gods, did the same to his warriors.

This prejudice, this inequality of gender reward, was not confined to the gods. Created by the Romans in 450 BC, the twelve tables were a set of conservative laws based on the traditional values, morals and beliefs of the early Roman society. They were often harsh. They declared females should remain in guardianship because of their levity of mind, even when they had attained their majority. Women were not allowed to drink and could not have the keys to the wine cellar in case they weakened and lost their 'purity', threatening the male's heritage. If found out, they could be put to death.

In the Americas, Itzamna was the creator god of the Mayans, father of the Bacabs, who upheld the corners of the world, and Huitzilopochtli was the patron god of the Aztecs, both civilizations offering an afterlife. For China, Shangti, also known as the Jade Emperor, was the supreme deity of creation, inviting departed kings to join him in the afterlife.

In the Judeo-Christian and Islamic monotheistic traditions, Yahweh, God or Allah, was very clearly the father and ordained man to have dominion over all creatures. He punished Adam and Eve for eating the forbidden fruit and proclaimed woman should be subordinate to man, and man must work and sweat for subsistence. The reward was to join Him in heaven.

The ethic of millennia of rural harmony and natural change

was replaced by the overwhelming and violent quest for conquest and for control and dominion over nature, animals and women. As man was given permission to rise above nature, it also provided social sanction to emphasise the moral worth of the individual, valuing independence and self-reliance. This freedom would open up to innovation and eventually lead to the rapid growth of science and technology.

The arms' race over the centuries that accompanied this expansion led to the full ugliness of war, with revolution continually introducing better weaponry and technology. The hideousness of war is always accompanied by the genius of innovation and invention. Without this arms' race, it is noted, there would never have been a trade-off for some beneficial side effects flowing to community, for example, faster communication (eg, the modern computer owes much to the genius of Second World War codebreaker Alan Turing at the cypher school at Bletchley Park), better transport and improved health systems. It is also noted that even though war was inextricably bound up with the rise of patriarchy, homo belli, this man of war, for all his destructiveness, had the spirit to offer the "supreme" sacrifice to protect those he loved in a less than perfect world. As Sam Keen has stated, Mars and Eros have always gone hand in hand.

We fight for dominance over territory, food, money, women, religion, ideological differences, anything. Even though there are now fewer wars than at any time in the past, wars will still be used to settle differences for many centuries yet. Whether using men, guns, planes, bullets, nuclear bombs, biological warfare or the Cybernet as weapons, we will always need to be prepared for war.

We should not be too surprised at this propensity for violence.

Some of this hereditary cargo can be clearly seen in our close cousins, the chimpanzees, with whom we share 98.6 per cent of our DNA.

Zarin Machanda, a primatologist at Tufts University, notes that chimps are jealous, selfish xenophobes and warmongers. Intercommunity combat is chaos. 'It is blood thirst. It is kill, kill, kill.' Even within communities, chimps commit ferocious acts of violence.

At no stage do they deem other monkeys as deserving of mercy or other moral considerations. Author Carl Sagan comments, 'They may be heroic in defending their own young, but they do not show the least compassion to the young of other species.'

It would seem violence is part of our nature but commentators are confident we can change. Machanda notes no other species matches us for kindness, compassion and empathy. She believes we can rise above our primal instincts.

In the earliest societies, the adage of the Roman general Vegetuis, 'If you want peace, prepare for war', was used to attest that one of the most effective means to ensure peace is always to be armed and ready to defend oneself. And by extension, while walking in the jungle, be armed for animal predators, although this was always going to be an unequal arms' race. As war was considered to be the normal state, eternal and inevitable, peace was simply described as a break between wars, not the other way around.

From the youngest age, boys gravitated to such toys as sticks and spears and were taught warfare, how to fight, how to kill, how to use weapons, in essence, how to be the victor. Even in modern sport, the saying 'Winning isn't everything; it's the only thing', attributed to UCLA Bruins football coach Henry Russell, is now a mantra for most elite sportspeople. Basically, like those schoolboy initiation ceremonies, sport was invented as a method to train for warfare. A modern coach will grasp this concept as a validation to use sport as a metaphor for life, without the need to actually kill or maim.

War is ugly and brutal, as are certain sports, and this is the dilemma a sensitive man faces. In a less than perfect world, the warrior can never wholly retire. It takes a balance of gentleness and fierceness to structure a whole man. Sport can fulfil these requirements. Some of the most competitive sports, whether they be football, boxing, basketball, tennis or golf, often require brutal aggression. Yet, between contests, most of these sportspeople can be the most gentle, affable and compassionate individuals. However, if necessary, a man or woman can now take the extra step to prepare for "war".

The philosophy of 'play up and play the game' still prevails as a mark of true sportsmanship or sportswomanship. I admire and appreciate healthy competitive sport. In my career as a sports and exercise physiotherapist, I have witnessed and officiated at hundreds of exciting, interesting and often spectacular sporting events. I encountered many character-building moments as competitors learned to deal with winning and losing.

As the inaugural physiotherapist for the Wallabies (Australia's national rugby union team) and the Kangaroos (the national rugby league team), and after attending many elite international cricket, basketball, soccer, surf life-saving and hockey events, as well as athletic and Commonwealth Games, I formed the opinion that sport is a metaphor for life. The remarkable and positive effects which radiate from the culture and infrastructure around sport enhance all aspects of life. Exercise, of itself, is a great lifestyle regulator in a modern society largely defined by sitting and inactivity.

Regardless, I don't condone sports which target and attack the head or the brain, such as boxing, and other such martial 'arts', a euphemism if ever there was one.

Essentially, whereas I clearly encourage competition, including controlled aggressive competition, I feel the old belligerent feather has been plucked a thousand times and a totally new feather is emerging. Intelligent thought and the inclination to read and acquiesce our emotions and feelings have revealed a new perspective, the way to a new feather, one I fully endorse.

CHAPTER THREE

The Uncommunicative Feather

*'I spent fifty per cent of my money on alcohol, women and gambling,
The other half I wasted,'*
WC Fields

It is a reasonable observation that men tend to use language assertively and are more likely to suppress or hold back their emotions. Women appear to have a wider-range of emotional vocabulary, using language more readily to describe their feelings and emotional states.

Recent research has shown it takes men an average of seven times longer to process high-intensity verbal communication than women. These differences can very easily lead to a perception that men are poor communicators.

With clear hindsight, and no apologies, it was fairly obvious now that in these early years, I was morphing into the typical male stereotype character.

As mentioned earlier, up to Grade 8 (thirteen years old) I attended a one-teacher school in a small rural community where my male role-models were independent and resilient farmers. The farms were mainly dairy and peanut-growing. Life was always full on. In winter, my father would wake about 4.30 am and start a fire in the kitchen stove as there was no electricity. He then went into the frost-covered fields, lead the cows into the bails and milk them. Next, he fed the pigs (in the piggery) and, after breakfast, attended to the rest of the farm, ploughing, fencing, repairs – whatever needed to be done. At 3 pm, he called the cows in again and repeated the process of milking. It was a relentless and tough existence.

Most of the farmers had served in the Second World War and gone through the Depression – they were hardened already by life. I could see this is what men did – this was our lot.

For the next four years I boarded at a boys-only college and my influence there was mainly from male teachers and boarding masters, also most them Second World War veterans.

When I finished senior school (Grade 12), I took three gap years to work out a career for myself. In this time, I duly fulfilled the rites of passage in the way males did in those days. I was introduced to alcohol, girls, sport and cars.

As soon as school was over, along with most of my year, I escaped for the traditional holiday at Surfers Paradise (now called 'Schoolies Week'). Besides what you expect may happen when a group of testosterone-driven young males and unchaperoned females meet for an unfettered week of fun heralding our release into the world, the most (un)memorable incident for me, came on the first Saturday night when I learned about the effects of alcohol in excess. I became paralytic – on vodka.

I regretted that either I was not advised this may happen or I chose not to listen to it. Very poor communication.

It wasn't easy for me to chart a career path. Initially, Dad was keen for me to apply for a position in the public service, the banks or insurance companies. After the harshness and instability of the Depression years before the war and the war years themselves, this was thought to be the ideal career for children of my parents' generation – security, regular pay, difficult to get sacked, great retirement benefits. So, I applied to all these institutions and waited for replies. After a few false starts, I eventually landed a job in the Queensland public service, selected to start work at the Repatriation Department.

This job was what I needed. Everybody was pleased, including my parents. The department looked after the affairs of war veterans. Over the course of the next three years, I would learn how "big business" worked. Starting in the registry and filing section, then learning how to write business letters, continuing on to meeting, understanding and gaining empathy with Diggers, to looking after their medical needs and helping with their pensions and entitlements.

I worked at hospitals, mainly the Repatriation General Hospital (RGH) at Greenslopes, the Tuberculosis Institute at Kenmore and the Rehabilitation Artificial Limb Appliance Centre (RALAC) at Windsor. I learnt how hospitals worked, how government worked and observed doctors and the medical profession at close quarters.

However, what pleased me just as much was the large staff social network. About 2000 personnel worked in these institutions, including at branch office in the city, of which probably 500 were young women. (In those days, the gender inequality meant that when women married they had to leave the public service). The rest were mainly Second World War veterans and a crop of younger clerks like me coming through as the new wave.

There was a tremendous social life within the department, with regular parties, sports functions and outings. We often mixed with the larger public service fraternity outside and life was really very exciting. I developed a great group of friends, was never short of a girlfriend or mate and generally grew in outlook on all matters.

Earlier in the first year, I began boxing training at the Police Citizens Youth Club at Lang Park, where Suncorp Stadium now sits. Queensland's best boxers were attracted here to train under Reg Layton. Reg had a stable of national and world champions and I attended the gym to train two or three times a week.

Boxing is such a basic, primitive and exciting endorphin event, it sits at the core of male culture – the Protect part of the 3 Ps. It is our martial identity and signals that this man is top of the gene pool. However, as we approach gender equality, many now consider this behaviour largely irrelevant as a means of conflict resolution and for attracting the opposite sex. The way I see the change in perspective with gender roles, I suspect the more modern "vulnerable" man and the "geek"' are now possibly viewed as top of the gene pool.

The other rite of passage that occurred in that year was that I bought my first car. There is almost no greater love than the first car – implying freedom and status. My choice of car was influenced by the *Silver Jacket* magazines I read as a teenager. There was a *Boys Own Paper* English journal which reported on all things masculine: soccer, horse racing, boxing, motor car and boat racing etc. I chose a 1949 MG-TC. It was fabulous. It was painted in British racing green and the sides of the motor cover were discarded to reveal a flashing platinum motor and carburettor. The bonnet was kept down by a trendy thick leather belt. It gave a throaty roar, hugged close to the ground and I felt like a million pounds roaring along with my peak cap on. (This was before our monetary system changed to dollars).

However, it was too expensive to run. I drove it hard and it often broke down. After five months I really couldn't afford it, so I begrudgingly sold it. Delusion over!

The Queensland Public Service had a very competitive rugby league competition and Repat supplied a strong team. I did well in this game. As a winger, I could use my speed to advantage. I was the highest points scorer for the three seasons I played with them, and in my second and third year I was selected for the Combined Public Service team.

However, by the third year at Repat, the fun aspect was diminishing as I realised that career wise, I was stagnating. Fun didn't make up for the lack of progress – or purpose. I gained the impression that the average public servant of this era had lost motivation by the time they were thirty, were devoid of challenge and became established in the system, cloaked in mediocrity. I started to find ways to extricate myself. By this stage, I had saved up enough to put myself through university.

While working at hospitals, I had seen and admired the work of the medical profession, so I enrolled at the University of Queensland to study physiotherapy.

I graduated as a physiotherapist in 1966 and almost immediately became married and started in private practice at the same time. There were no such entities as life coaches in this era and my university course didn't educate about business acumen, finance management, work-life balance or personal health. Nor did it teach about the need to communicate, or even how to communicate. I was simply armed with energy, enthusiasm, optimism and hope.

At this stage, physiotherapists were not generally involved with treating sportspeople. However, because I was still an active sportsperson, my practice quickly attracted patients from all sports, particularly the contact sports and football codes. I co-founded Sports Medicine in Queensland in 1970 and my practice thrived.

So much so, that in 1977, after ten years of intense engagement, teaching, learning and being constantly stimulated, I was beginning to burn out – to run down. I regularly worked in the evenings and officiated at two or three games over a weekend. During these years I witnessed and supervised hundreds of exciting and often spectacular sporting events. This included attending many riveting rugby clashes against the All Blacks, Lions, Pumas and the Springboks as well as Commonwealth Games and World Games.

I had the privilege of being involved with motivated and talented elite athletes of all sports of that era. In the process, I witnessed many outstanding and inspirational performances. However, by now, I had seen so many football games and so many sporting events, I was becoming jaded with them.

My health was suffering. I felt overwhelmed, extremely tired and defeated. I was losing perspective, growing cynical and fantasising about throwing in my job. I was becoming uncommunicative, a set of circumstances which were reflected in my personal relationships. In reality, I was suffering from a form of burn-out, a term not officially used in those days and not recognised then as a medical condition.

What was going on here?

From the earliest days, boys were taught that they must have a career. They must have a valid vocation, a means to survive and provide for themselves, their family, their tribe and extended community. They are taught it is a manly thing to do, to spend long days in the field, hunting, ploughing, milking cows, mustering. Or choose demanding careers in medicine, law, music, the arts, business, engineering, or any of the trades etc. Work has become a defining aspect of man's existence.

Since the Industrial Revolution, with advancements in widespread technology, men, and women have become chained to assembly lines, doing shiftwork at night, running massive factories and mines, building houses or cleaning toilets. The recent advent of the technological and IT revolution, leading to AI (artificial intelligence), otherwise rational men are spending longer time locked in a desk and chair, addictively producing work by staring at a computer screen for eight hours or more. This can become a heroic backbreaking life, mundane and devoid of joy and humour, supressing opportunities for riotous fun and exploring Peter Pan and other adventurous outbursts.

Zorba said it best: 'A man needs a touch of madness otherwise he will never be free.' Scratch the surface of a rational man, you will find a wild man waiting to be freed.

This blinkered focus has often been shown to lead to an unbalanced view of life, limiting opportunities for healthy lifestyles. The so-called "successful" executive works up to seventy hours a week and rises high in the organisation on a handsome salary, while his marriage and family fall apart. His health declines, he may smoke and drink too heavily, and lives only for his work.

This lifestyle can prevent fathers from having a strong and positive influence on their children, sharing role-making decisions and being significantly involved in their life. This strong masculine ethic involving stereotypical stress-relieving rowdy beers at the end of the day, discussing football, cars and sex, also strengthens opportunities to reinforce misogynist dogmatism, easily dismissing men who are intuitive, sensitive and artistic (wusses). In reality, most modern men are more complex than this. They, in fact, demand more, but many struggle to break free.

Chapter Three The Uncommunicative Feather

The cruel irony is that this lifestyle impacts on his relationship with his partner – the one he is working hard to support. The one he must communicate with. To understand this disconnect, we must look at the other aspect which defines man's existence – woman. Men's initial experience of a woman is that with his mother, the Earth Mother. He will view her as a vehicle enabling him to justify his own mortality and existence. There is an 1884 song,

> A boy's best friend is his mother,
> Cherish her with care
> And smooth her silver hair,
> For when she's gone, you'll get no other.
> (Miller and Skelley).

Further, it is important to acknowledge the influence that our mothers may have exerted on the way we see ourselves. Even before we had language, she wordlessly taught us trustworthiness and security, fulfilled our desires for satisfaction for food and warmth. We also learned judgement, disappointment, anger and fear from the reflection of her face and from her cradled arms. If she is tense or fearful, we could also learn the world could be tense and dangerous through her emotions. Her body and reactions to life situations are our first information system. By her attitudes, we are subconsciously programmed for life for many of our habits, traits and fears, good and bad. Later, she is the prime teacher of social skills, personal hygiene, style and relationships and manners. We are taught to be prepared for all occasions, just in case 'the queen comes to dinner.' (Or recently, the king).

At the same time, our fathers were generally background

figures forging security and stability. Someone from whom we silently learned by osmosis and actions, more than words.

On the one hand, such as how to respect a woman but also how to react to displeasure, by either calm or anger, such as road rage, domestic violence, etc.

The second aspect relating to woman is the erotic or sexual force, the magnet that most men can be irresistibly attracted to, and a circumstance in which males are responsive to women. This is a seeming paradox. Even though it appears that men are the dominant gender, when it comes to attraction, women are, in reality, the prime movers. He may think he initiates, but her inspiring beauty and pheromones draws him to her. And she does the selecting.

Amir Livine is a psychiatrist interested in "attachment". In his 2020 book *Attached*, he says soulmates are possible because of the neurocircuitry in our brains. For humans, research has shown appearance is an important part of how we pick our mates – visual first, then smell, body odour and pheromones, oxytocin and vasopressin.

Witness a beautiful woman wearing a stunning gown as she makes an entrance. Most men in the room will spontaneously swivel to gaze at the vision. Some experienced men will resist, offering a fleeting glance, her presence impossible to ignore, but then feign to dismiss her; others will intently stare like a deer caught in the glare of headlights. These men will be mysteriously mesmerised, intimidated even, triggering off a deep primeval yearning response. Artists have long recognised this phenomenon, allowing such beautiful arias as *Silent Worship* from Handel's 1728 opera *Ptolemy*, to be created.

> Did you not hear My Lady
> Go down the garden singing
> Blackbird and thrush were silent
> To hear the alleys ringing...
> Oh, saw you not My Lady,
> Out in the garden there?
> Shaming the rose and the lily
> For she is twice as fair.
> Though I am nothing to her
> Though she must rarely look at me
> And though I could never woo her
> I love her till I die.

This song suggests the admirer is attracted to her beauty. The truth is, it's about lust; lust inspired by physical cues.

This automatic response is wired into our hard drive, encoded millions of years ago. If one of our early, ancient vertebrate ancestors either noticed, or received, an encouraging message (or not), from an amenable female, he had maybe a fraction of a second to act, to beat either a potential competitor or a predator.

This aspect of woman, the sexual woman, exudes a mysticism that is difficult to resist, attracting men of all types, from creative artists to the addictive workers. For many men, the woman unleashes the creative drive and inspiration for their life, their work, their creativity, whether it be painting, sculpture, architecture, building an empire, or even to climbing the highest mountain, or sometimes to motivate deeds of criminality.

Regarding this primeval sense of attraction to a beautiful woman, even though beauty is clearly in the eyes of the beholder, anthropologists and sociologists tend to agree that the primary focus for a male is to unconsciously register the ratio of waist to hips. This must be 0 to 0.4. Consistent in every race, whether tall like Scandinavians, shorter like Asians, larger like Polynesians, or whether individually they are overweight or skinny, a man's innate experience will draw him towards this important ratio of 0 to 0.4, reflecting child-bearing hips.

This can be strengthened by personal cultural and local fashionable proclivities concerning posture, leg length and shape, breast size, hair style and eyebrow shapes. These can all change within a season, a decade or a generation. It is now clearly recognised that facial attractiveness played a major role in shaping evolution. The Natural History Museum in August 2007 stated studies on our fossil ancestors have shown our choice of sexual partners has shaped the human face.

Men with large jaws, flaring cheeks and large eyebrows were seen to be sexy, in the eyes of our ancestors. As well, many scientific reviews show that adult faces of males and females with high baby schema have been rated as more attractive.

Moreover, adult female faces with a high level of baby schema elicit caretaking behaviour. And both genders are initially attracted to the opposite sex who have youngish-looking baby faces, large eyes, full lips, small chin, features which are considered to imply warmth, trust, cooperation and helplessness, and elicit a "cuteness" response. You could be describing a baby or a supermodel.

The same force, at the other end of the spectrum, also inspires a particular type of man to believe it is his right to cross boundaries, to control, to use force and commit violence and sexual assault. They take no responsibility for their actions, blaming the woman, attributing her raw beauty and subliminal messages – 'It was her fault, she wore provocative clothing, she smiled at me and seduced me.' He has cruelly been subjected to primal hijack.

At many levels, I concede it would be helpful if men could improve their communication skills. Generally, men are solution-oriented individuals who go into problem-solving mode when met with a challenge. My experience is that I could do this better by becoming a better listener and not jumping in. It is important to see all sides of a situation.

I also learned that it is important to learn how to communicate, to seek advice, to study, discuss pertinent issues in society and make meaningful friendships.

Recently, I have observed an almost tectonic shift in men's ability to effectively listen, to share problems, to communicate appropriately and who are reshaping this feather.

CHAPTER FOUR

The Repugnant Feather – Domestic Violence

This is the feather which is the most odious of all. It is the one which should be plucked as soon as possible. And it is not only the male who may reveal this plumage.

While violence and abuse strike couples of all races, religions, socio-economic status and sexual orientations, the risk factors for women or men becoming victims of abusers include having a partner with traditional beliefs that they have the right to control their other half. With males, this often follows one of the themes of this book, the belief that women are not equal to men.

A recent Australian study found that men's belief in traditional male stereotypes has a stronger effect than other key demographic indicators on their likelihood of being violent.

A survey of 1000 young Australian men found the belief that men should be breadwinners, or should act tough, is twenty-five times more accurate in predicting violence than education, address or cultural background.

The study, titled *Unpacking the Man Box* was undertaken by Jesuit Social Services and Dr Michael Flood of the Queensland University of Technology. The report showed masculine stereotypes stop young men living healthy lives and being their best selves.

The executive director of Jesuit Social Services, Matt Tyler, said, 'This report demonstrates the significant costs of young men and others of being "in the man box"' – meaning they personally endorse a range of behaviours related to rigid gender roles, aggression, control and acting tough. These stereotypes have unique powerful influences on harmful attitudes and behaviours.'

Witness the recent television documentary concerning schoolboys at a prestigious Melbourne boys' school, singing a chant on a packed train, 'I wish that all the ladies were holes in the road/ if I was a dump truck/I'd fill them with my load.' Every line is immersed in learned misogynous behaviour.

There are other reasons. Abusers may also feel the need to control their partner because of low self-esteem, extreme jealousy, difficulties in regulating anger and other strong emotions, or when they feel inferior to their partner in education and socio-economic background. Other risk factors include poverty and lack of a high school education, plus alcohol.

Alcohol and drugs may also contribute to violent behaviour, so it makes sense for certain individuals to keep drink and drug use to a minimum. And some fundamentalist religious teachings may also have a case to answer.

A percentage of men may have an undiagnosed personality disorder or psychological disorder. Still, others may have learned this behaviour from growing up in a household where domestic violence was accepted as a normal part of being raised in their family. They may have seen violence often or they may have been victims themselves.

What is important in the context of this book is that boys who learn that women are not to be valued or respected and who see violence directed against women, are more likely to abuse women when they grow up. For these men, this is a learned experience.

Just as importantly, the question is often asked,: why do women stay in abusive relationships? Unfortunately, this can have the effect of shaming, blaming or holding the victim responsible for the abuser's actions. Judgement by social media can often be harsh in this regard. One such response inspired American domestic violence researchers Jaclyn Cravens, Jason Whiting and Rolo Aamar to identify key reasons women remain in abusive relationships. Editor Kylie Lang reports on these findings:

> Distorted thoughts are one. Being hurt and controlled can be traumatising and give rise to doubts and self-blame. A victim can be so worn down and anxious they believe they deserve the abuse, or somehow triggered it.
>
> Fear is another. The threat of physical and emotional harm is powerful and female victims are more likely than male victims to be terrorised and traumatised.
>
> Some women hope to save their partner by loving them enough to "fix them and teach them kindness".
>
> Mothers can sacrifice their own safety to protect their children from abuse or because they think it is vital their kids have a dad present.
>
> Family expectations and experiences factor in it too. If a woman saw her father beat her mother, that can normalise the abuse. It is what love looks like.
>
> Others stay for financial reasons, including debt racked up in their name by their hostile partner.
>
> Some women, the researchers found, are threatened by isolation.

After being deliberately separated from their family and friends by their controlling abuser, they wonder if they can ever rejoin their loved ones.

For some women, often multiple presentations of the above apply, creating a nasty dysfunctional situation, particularly if substance abuse is included.

No cause of domestic violence justifies the actions of the abuser, nor should any cause be used as a rationale for their behaviour. Understanding and acknowledging these possible causes may help an abuser realise it is not acceptable to abuse their partner physically, sexually, psychologically or emotionally, particularly by coercive means.

Coercive violence (or control) is a particularly sinister, insidious mode of abuse and dominating behaviour. The perpetrator (usually a male), may do things such as monitor their partner's phone, isolate them from friends and family, limit access to finances, humiliate and cyberstalk them and seek to control aspects of who they are and how they live their life. They "gaslight" them, the modern term for the act of undermining another person's reality by denying facts, the environment around them, or their feelings.

Some of the answers to manage domestic violence may be found by introducing this new feather in the next chapter.

Having stated this, the Australian Bureau of Statistics has released new insights into coercive control, or emotional abuse. It reports nearly as many men as women say their current partners have tried to control their contact with family, friends or people in the community. These insights were pulled from the Personal Safety Survey in 2016. The bureau also said emotional abuse increased between the ages of thirty and forty-four for men and women.

There are no excuses.

As a civilised society, we must declare domestic violence to be inadmissible, repugnant and cowardly. It is important that we listen and we offer assistance. Ultimately, these males will need to change their behaviour. Good men are urged to make a stand and reach out to mates who appear vulnerable. Ask, 'Are you okay?' instead of thinking, 'It's not my business.'

Men are consistently often slow to move to help another man. Too often as men, we have spent our lives jumping in with solutions to other people's challenges, but often we feel inadequate to assist men with mental health issues. The reality is, you don't need to fix someone, all you need to do is to be there to support them.

CHAPTER FIVE

The Exemplar Feather – Be a Positive Role Model

'Being a role model is the most powerful form of educating – youngsters need good models more than they need critics. It's one of a parent's greatest responsibilities and opportunities,' – John Wooden, US basketball player and coach. Values can't simply be taught as a list of instructions; they need to be seen and lived and embedded through actions. 'Boys will not respect girls because they are told it is the right thing to do,' says Australian columnist, TV and radio commentator and author Angela Mollard. 'They learn through how their father treats their mother, and a waitress and his female colleagues.'

So, we need to continue to be inspirational figures in our teen's lives. They learn these skills at the dinner table and family and social functions. Boys learn by seeing, by experiencing real men who are happy, healthy, enjoy their work and their relationships. Encourage them not to be influenced by the ones they see on television, film, social media or the news. These are not necessarily good or real men.

The sex lives of teens became a national conversation in 2021 when former student Chanel Contos posed a question on Instagram, 'Have you or a close friend been sexually assaulted by someone who went to an all-boys' school in Sydney?'

Within twenty-four hours, 204 people had responded 'yes', prompting the then 22-year-old to set up a website which, three weeks later, had garnered 6000 testimonies. Contos started a petition demanding consent classes in schools and a year after her first Instagram post, education ministers unanimously agreed to mandate consent education in schools from 2022.

There is also an opportunity for boys to be positive role models for other boys. I have had discussions with mothers of 15-, 16- and 17-year-old boys who when they examine their boys' mobile phones despair at the degree of derogatory language their sons use in relation to females.

There is no marshalling of this cyberspace culture and peer pressure insists this is the standard boys adhere to in order to be accepted. Fundamental change is needed in this society. As mentioned, school-based programs are helpful as are discussions at home with parents. However, the real secret to changing an unacceptable culture may lie within values young people bring to these groups.

You would be hard pressed to find a better example of a young man championing this change than Mason Black. Mason was the school captain at Brisbane Boys' College when he presented a powerful speech to his peers in March 2021 in relation to domestic violence. It was widely featured in the media at large after the initial report in Brisbane's *Courier Mail*:

> The narrative needs to change. Boys, it feels like no matter where we look, this issue is not at the forefront of everyone's mind, but why not?
> What you really need is a basic acceptance and respect, and

that, boys, is on all of us. Boys, if a woman wants to say no, and she says no, we have to listen, understand and accept this. As good as this message is when coming from public speakers or staff, it's up to us. The boys.

It makes me feel sick and it makes me feel embarrassed that our school is featured in the testimonies of young women who are victims of sexual assault, he said, referring to a recent national report by hundreds of female victims.

If you have ever objectified a woman based on her looks, talked about females in a misogynistic way, or taken advantage without consent, you are part of the problem.

Stop being boys, be human.

This starts with putting an end to slurs and derogatory comments about women.

We have to keep our mates accountable, no matter where it may be.

Mason made many other points concerning empowering women to live a life without fear, for women to wear what they want without judgment, and that they feel supported.

Within three days, Mason's speech had gone viral and, in that time, had more than 300,000 views on Instagram alone.

Noting the response to Mason's speech, this is an ideal place to acknowledge the strength of social media, and to heighten our awareness of its ability to influence, positively and negatively. This is an opportunity to scrutinise and perhaps identify the meaningless things to which the media may have given meaning, such as certain narcissistic social media sites.

Be wary of video games. For children, there are some marvellous skills to be learned here. Most games are attractive to boys and girls almost equally as they offer a challenge that is often to some degree puzzle based, with exciting characters, colours and sounds. The content is extremely safe, and such games provide an opportunity to develop memory, problem solving skills, challenges, patience, fast thinking and resilience. At this stage, excluding only the benefits of sun, fresh air and exercise, it is hard to criticise games with any real conviction.

After the age of fourteen, adult themes are found more and more in games. Violence, gore and guns are the dominant features of these. Studies suggest that some of the most popular video games are disengaging boys and men from the real world. Another study reported that thirty-one per cent of males and thirteen per cent of females felt addicted to video games. Most video games are variations on war games and encourage violence, the winner being the one who can kill more of the "enemy". The player must always keep their vision on what is reality. In real life once you are dead, you are dead; you don't get another chance as you do on a video game.

Along these same lines, be critical and vocal about pornography. Viewing online pornography is routine, especially among young men and boys. As Michael Sheather, associate editor of the *Australian Women's Weekly*, reported in the December 2020 edition, fifty-three per cent of boys have viewed pornography by age thirteen. This is reinforced by a recent report from the Australian Institute of Families where studies found about half of all children aged nine to sixteen had regular exposure to porn, boys more likely to deliberately seek it out. As a recent review of forty-three studies among adolescents and emerging adults documents, sexually explicit and sexually violent media have clear effects on domestic and sexual violence perpetration and victimisation. Michael Flood, from the law faculty of the Queensland University of Technology, stated pornography teaches sexist and sexually objectifying understandings of gender and sexuality.

Young Australians are contending with a powerful porn industry drugging our kids with hardcore, violent sexual material. The content has been shown to degrade women, normalise rape and sexual violence, and can enforce gender stereotypes.

Easy access to pornography means boys often spend years watching graphic sexual acts, which rarely feature consent, communication or condoms, before engaging in sexual activity. Rachel Hinds, a manager for Top Blokes, a mental health program charity tailored for boys, states, 'Boys have a four or five-year education on what love, sex and intimacy looks like through high levels of high-violence porn. It teaches them that women enjoy being degraded and treated as an object.'

Clearly it shapes how boys and men see girls and women, and how girls and women see themselves. A recent survey found that young men did not know that women had pubic hair and were shocked. This is because women are clean shaven in pornography.

Adolescents need to know porn stars aren't meant to look real. Dr Harold Koplewicz, president of the Child Mind Institute, relates, 'Many of those bodies are surgically exaggerated and further exaggerated by the way they are styled and photographed. Porn sex isn't real – it's fantasy.'

In a randomised experimental study among young adults in Denmark, exposure to (nonviolent) pornography led to less egalitarian attitudes and higher levels of hostile sexism among young men. In a longitudinal study among US adolescents, increased use of sexually explicit media predicted more sexist attitudes for girls two years later.

Further, pornography teaches sexually aggressive and violence-supported behaviours. Correlational studies also found associations between pornography and actual violent behaviours. Men who use pornography more often are more likely to practise or desire dominant and degrading practices, such as gagging and choking.

Just as disturbingly, women who use pornography are more likely to practise or desire submissive practices such as being choked, slapped or gagged.

However, the effects of pornography need not be inevitable or all-powerful. The impacts of pornography are mediated by four factors: the characteristics of the viewer, their engagement with the material, its content, and the character and context of use. Sexual and domestic violence is shaped by multiple social and cultural factors, of which pornography use is only one.

As counsellor Chris Brett-Renes notes, we should think of pornography like we do alcohol. Both have the potential to be harmful but for most people, occasional use isn't a cause for concern. However, as with alcohol, pornography can be used as a coping mechanism or lead to addiction.

Pornography use can also contribute to problems with sexual function, including erectile problems or delayed ejaculation. If a man watches hours of porn and masturbates frequently, his penis can become less sensitive. Rather than go without, he may start to grip his penis harder to achieve sufficient stimulation – a "death grip". This has the contradictory effect of further reducing sensitivity, making it gradually even more difficult to reach orgasm.

To reduce the harms to children and young people, it is vital that comprehensive sexuality education with alternative and age-appropriate content be provided by parents and in schools. It has been suggested sex education should be mandated as part of the curriculum from primary school onwards. There should be funding for specialists to go into schools to have those difficult conversations. Regardless, talking about sex and pornography must start in the family. Talk about it with your children. This should be a community project.

Instead of having them search for pornography, encourage young men to learn something else – seek education. At their fingertips, their keyboard, they have access to an unlimited and ever increasing well of information. They can find courses and e-books or real books, so they can learn about the history of the world, the universe, back to the "big bang". The *Time-Life* series is an excellent place to start to learn about great leaders, innovations, music, the arts and science. Search for inspirational and adventurous stories and characters.

Call out behaviour; be a witness. We must start calling out any male who we know has perpetrated any type of domestic violence. One of the most critical steps here is to be committed to addressing family and domestic violence. Most authorities believe that this must be addressed in the context of gender equality. All forms of violence in society warrants condemnation and it is important to place violent behaviour in the context of other political, legal and social responses aimed at ending gender-based inequalities. The long-term prevention of male family violence requires a clear and consistent message from all individuals and social providers. All forms of violence are unacceptable and won't be tolerated.

As previously mentioned, domestic violence is not the prerogative of males dominating females as recent reports quote a high percentage of women are violent towards their partners.

Men and women need to know their use of violence will not be condoned by any person or institution. They need to see that everyone, including individuals, community providers, police and the legal system will protect the rights of others to safety.

It is important to recognise that men who use violence to gain power and control with damaging effects to others, also report a range of damaging effects for themselves. These include shame, guilt, self-loathing and frustrations at not having the kinds of relationships with their partners and families they might like to have. Although it involves them giving up the use of power and control and the privileges of domination, men also have much to gain from learning to have equal, open and non-violent relationships.

This is a call for men to change on a number of levels, such as in their thinking, feelings, attitudes and behaviour. They may need to learn new skills, and to practice and integrate these in their lives, and recognise that the change process is gradual and takes time.

They should be offered support and encouragement to explore their behaviour and learn unfamiliar and sometimes confronting new ways of knowing themselves and others. At the same time, this may include accepting responsibility for their behaviour and being reminded when they fail to do so.

Men may need to recognise that feelings are different from behaviours and that there are achievable and variable alternatives to using violent and controlling behaviours. And to realise that such change is rarely involved with anger management, so not to get them confused. This is where an experienced counsellor may need to be sought. Start with a general practitioner, local police station or a respected counsellor.

Challenge stereotypes – yours and others. Change ingrained and rigid expectations and beliefs about sex-role stereotyping, about the roles of women and men such as women caring for the home and children, while men are the bread-winners.

Use language and actions that are respectful of women, encouraging equality in every aspect. This means particularly listening and sharing conversations and sharing decision-making. Be wary of put-down and demeaning language, including unwitting condescension and dismissiveness. This form of overt unconscious bias and unintentional prejudice is often at the hands of otherwise well-meaning and decent men. Unconscious bias is where your background, personal experiences, societal stereotypes and cultural context influence your decisions and actions without you realising. This behaviour undermines confidence. If you experience another male, or person of any gender, acting in this way, approach them and gently explain the need to change. The standard you walk past is the standard you accept. The attitude is so often ingrained, they generally don't realise they are doing this. If you don't tell them, they may never know. When Oprah Winfrey was asked to state the greatest hurdle she had overcome, she answered, 'The disease to please. It happens when we are not raised to know our own value and our own worth.'

This follows a powerful quote attributed to Eleanor Roosevelt, 'No one can make you feel inferior without your consent.'

Following on from this, changes in social attitudes over the past few decades have made it easier to give offence in many ways, particularly with speech, intentionally or unintentionally.

There are many different areas requiring respect to personal characteristics, not solely to women, or gender identity or gender expression. The list includes race, colour, religion, pregnancy, national origin, ancestry, citizenship status, age, marital status, physical disability, mental disability, medical condition and military or veteran status.

As languages historian Professor Rollo Sussex notes, there is an old Australian custom of robust larrikin humour which calls on some categories in the above list. Intention is important. Some statements can be taken as disrespectful when they are intended to be jocular. Sussex impresses you cannot rely on intention as a rationale. This list is receiver oriented and what matters most is how the receiver interprets it. It is safest when you talk to or about your peers. It is risky to make jokes or speak disparagingly, or even ambiguously, about people from other groups than your own. Don't say things that can be misinterpreted – think carefully about the effect of your words on others.

Be particularly wary of quick throwaway lines you may post on social media – these can be easily misinterpreted.

The exemplar feather is obviously one we should aspire to acquire, and nurture. In reality, it may look unruffled or perfect, but in fact it is executing the best values of mankind.

CHAPTER SIX

The Creative Feather

'A vision without strategy remains an illusion,'
— Lee Bolman

After graduation from university, I raced headlong into my life with nothing more than my wife sitting beside me, my diploma, hope, creativity burning inside me, and a great deal of confidence.

I say this as an acknowledgment that peacocks are often associated with confidence, exhibiting their beautiful feathers without fear of judgment or rejection. This is a good feather.

However, after intensely working hard for ten years I began suffering from a form of burnout. Not knowing how to manage this, I considered walking away from my career. However, I decided I should take a break, have some time off and reassess my position and priorities. I suspected I needed a plan for a different, healthier lifestyle.

So, with my wife and children aged nine and seven, I flew to England to begin an extended break. The plan was to tour through Europe in a van for six weeks.

On the way across, we had a week in Singapore so I could attend an international physiotherapy conference. It was timely and a game-changer for me. The guest speaker, Los Angeles psychologist Leo Buscaglia, spoke about love. Not religious or marital love, but personal love. This was "New Age" stuff back then. He put forward the idea that we should, as individuals, be more insightful, spend time to examine who we are, and search for and release the unique individual inside. Life is not all about empire building, power, money, sex or status – or ego.

That started me thinking. He finished by reading out a letter which appeared in the *Journal of Humanistic Psychology*. It was written by an eighty-five-year-old who was dying who wrote,

> If I had my life to live over again, I'd try to make more mistakes next time. I wouldn't try to be perfect. I would relax more. I'd limber up. I'd be sillier than I've been on this trip. I know very few things that I would take seriously. I'd be crazier. I'd be less hygienic. I'd take more chances. I'd take more trips. I'd climb more mountains. I'd swim more rivers, I'd watch more sunsets, and I'd go more places I've never been to. I'd travel. I'd eat more ice cream and less broccoli. I'd have more actual troubles and fewer imaginary ones.
>
> You see, I was one of those people who lived prophylactically and sensible and sanely, hour after hour, day after day. Oh, I've had my moments, but if I had to do it all over again, I would have nothing but beautiful moments – moment by moment by moment. I'm one of those people who never went anywhere without a thermometer, a hot water bottle, a raincoat and a parachute. If I had to do it all over again, I'd travel lighter next time. If I had to do it all over again, I'd start barefoot

earlier in the spring and stay that way later in the fall. I'd ride more merry-go-rounds. I'd watch more sunrises and I'd play with more children, if I had my life to live over again, but you see I don't.

The words resonated strongly with me. I was ready for them. In retrospect, I believe they were largely responsible for my addressing and changing my attitude towards life. There was no need for me to compete against the rest of the world – only myself.

On my return from Europe, I began to reassess my life's priorities. The first step was to redefine success. I came to understand that success cannot simply be measured by whether you win or lose. It is about realising your potential – not what you achieve or how you are judged or compared to somebody else.

To do this meant redesigning my life. The concept of planning a healthy lifestyle is not new; you win or lose. But in this era, the idea was never considered seriously important. I set out to manage my life as a total enterprise, much as you would manage a corporation – I designed a business plan.

The first key principle was to find balance. To do this meant searching for a low-stress lifestyle with a right proportion of work and play, of challenge and ease, of stress and relaxation, of striving and taking it easy, of companionship and solitude, of exercise and rest, of discipline and self-indulgence.

The goal was NOT to eliminate stress. Without stress, there is no challenge. The art was to get it to the level where it could assist me to enjoy a stimulating lifestyle. Simply, I found an effective lifestyle is based on the philosophy that human happiness, health and wellbeing are a holistic proposition. As I mentioned earlier, this implies that you cannot be effective in your business life, and unhealthy or ineffective in your private life, or in any other area of life. I reasoned that if I were to follow a single dream, such as becoming president of a company, or making a million dollars, achieving it may not live up to my expectations. There may be personal hidden costs that I did not expect on the way, with parts of myself remaining unfulfilled. Genuine success is not STATIC, therefore, but DYNAMIC. The concept of dynamic success appears difficult because it allows no absolute limits. It forces the individual to formulate his own limits, standards and values. In the end, this becomes a valuable exercise as it allows room for personal growth in all areas. To break the pattern of imbalance, I reviewed my life as an overall proposition and made some new decisions about how to invest time and energy. In this regard, I am reminded of Aristotle who believed true happiness comes only from a life of meaning – of doing what is worth doing.

Essentially, I constructed my lifestyle from six general areas of living. Let me expand on some of the six basic dimensions.

Professional: This is my means of livelihood and will be my life's central activity. It is vital that I like my job and derive satisfaction from it. I figured that if I didn't look forward to work every day, I would have either to change my attitude or change jobs.

Financial: This relates to money, material goods and possessions and things that give me feelings of security and satisfaction. Success in this area means developing saleable job skills, adequate money for my needs and security in case of ill health, recession or loss of job. It need not involve millions, but simply learning to live within one's budget.

Social: Relationships and activities that I share with others;

families, friends, members of the opposite sex. It is important that I belong to organisations or clubs to extend my interests. It is also important to associate with work colleagues socially, and join in recreational activities with other people – parties, theatre, picnics, etc.

Cultural: These are activities I do for rewarding educational purposes. They are self-broadening activities such as travelling, reading, studying a foreign language, taking courses for the sake of learning, attending lectures, watching educational television programs, going to plays, worthwhile movies, concerts and the theatre. It is the way in which I absorb new ideas, and expand my horizons in all different directions and enjoy learning new things.

Creative: This really means searching for the artist inside. These are activities which allow me to express my personality and which encourage growth. These include hobbies, crafts or artwork, painting, or sculpture, playing a musical instrument, gardening and growing flowers, building things, remodelling a home, singing, dancing or acting in a play or revue. This means any avenues for enjoying yourself by expressing your uniqueness. The burgeoning field of neuroasthetics examines the biological basis of our emotional responses to art. Research shows that engaging with art can activate the brain's reward system, releasing chemicals such as dopamine, serotonin and oxytocin.

Do not let the artist inside you die! Let it out.

Personal: Success in this area means being in sound health (mental and physical). This means exploring the wellness triad of rest, exercise and diet. It is important to recognise the mutually supporting synergistic relationship between these three factors. This section also included spiritual pursuits, privacy and self-understanding, emotional stability and personal adjustment. This included, for me, learning to meditate. Meditation produces chemicals that foster feelings of worth and belonging, as well as lowering stress levels caused by "busyness". It is one of the most evidence-based strategies for preventing burnout. It should not be dismissed. It needs to be done consistently to train your brain to get the benefit from it – every day

In effect, organising my life meant sitting down and deliberately planning a balanced approach. I learned to pigeonhole my day and week to ensure I made time to include all dimensions, including hobbies, creative outlets, social life, exercise, continuing education, family and time with children, plus personal time, relaxation, holidays for myself and a dedicated twenty minutes of meditation every day.

There is no silver bullet for this change. There was no hurry to do this. I added components of change, little by little over the years until I considered the change became effective. I was also aware that research has shown it can take up to three months to effectively change a behaviour.

American productivity expert Charles Duhigg adds, 'Changing one core habit can trigger a reaction that encourages you to change other habits.'

Over the years, I have continually updated attention to my lifestyle. However, as the next chapter reveals, part of this challenge was to confront and address "The Ivory Tower of Manhood".

CHAPTER SEVEN

The Denial Feather – the Ivory Tower of Manhood

An ivory tower is a metaphorical place, or an atmosphere, where people are cut off from the rest of the world in favour of their own pursuit. In this instance, it is men.

In our lifetime, women in the Western world have advanced in ways nearly unimaginable from when I was a boy. However, it is very clear that women are still trapped and oppressed in so many parts of the world, and subjugated to the dictates of men. But men are also trapped, in culturally defined roles. Witness the angst as they negotiate the slippery stairway to this ivory tower of manhood. Watching our sons being twisted into society's expectations of men can be frustrating and counterproductive. And guilt-laden when we don't address it as parents.

At first, it appears that male socialisation supports the case that the male's basic experience is the opposite of intimacy. We are not expected to be seen as vulnerable, to cry, or to show weakness of any sort. That is how we define ourselves. To illustrate this point, in 1996, when I was 52, I was diagnosed with prostate cancer after a routine blood (PSA) test.

The surgeon was gentle as he explained that without invasive treatment I may have three, perhaps five years left. The immediate shock was enormous. However, that night while sharing the news with my wife I didn't communicate the full story or my deepest fears. I put on my bravest face and calmly and methodically tried to put a positive spin on it.

It didn't work. The next morning, we drove over to a retailer to buy a new motor mower and on the way back home the full impact hit me. I suddenly jammed the car to a halt next to a park, hopped out and ran across the park. With no one around, I bawled unrestrainedly at the top of my voice. What was the point of buying a motor mower if I wasn't going to be here? What was the point of doing anything? The questions and scrutiny flowed furiously.

So, men do cry. And we are vulnerable. And we are not invincible. (More on prostate cancer later). It's not that difficult to imagine how this denial or resistance to seeking help eventuated. After all, our generation was spawned by an unbroken line of men who were imbued with the ideals of chivalry, a concept which began a thousand years ago, in Crusader days, with the onset of knighthood. These ideals proclaim men should aspire to be perfect gentlemen, faithful, courteous to women, pure, brave, stoic and fearless, unsparing of self, bowing before God and womankind – sentiments that today are considered by many to be worthy of disdain and largely irrelevant.

The actions of a chivalrous man towards a woman in the corporate world, the business world or the wider community could now generally be seriously rejected. The idea of opening the door for a woman, or pulling out her chair for her at a board meeting could immediately compromise the dynamics of the power balance. These actions could imply: 'you are a member of the "weaker sex",' evoking a sense to everybody in the room that the stronger male is going to be in charge here. At this level, women may not want to be seen to be accepting any degree of patriarchy, or chivalry. Simply, I believe the least they want are acknowledgements, empathy, respect and consideration. There is also a complication here with flirtatious behaviour, an often innate and unwitting "game" which can also be misread. Flirting, or coquetry, is social and sexual conduct involving spoken or written communication, as well as body language, by one person to another, either to suggest interest in a deeper relationship with the other person, or, if done playfully, for amusement. Or to unleash a more primeval relationship – to "mate".

The complication, or difficulty, is to ascertain the intention, whether the instigator simply wants to be friendly or wants to tease; or it may be a serious attempt to develop a more meaningful relationship.

Without knowing the other person's intentions, flirting and friendly behaviour are often nearly identical and this makes knowing the difference extremely frustrating for everyone involved, whether at work, socially or personally. At corporate or board room level, even subtle flirting is fraught; it can disadvantage either of the two people involved and be unsettling to other members witnessing the display. It is actually fraught everywhere and in many instances is deemed "inappropriate".

Such body language as holding strong eye contact (a very vital part of flirting, keeping in mind science reported the average optical non-flirting eye-contact is 3.3 seconds), flashing a gorgeous smile, offering a compliment, tilting your head forward, giving a light touch on the arm or hand, and playing with your hair. All these mannerisms are generally grouped as attention-seeking behaviours.

Away from the workplace, flirting can be fun, teasing and, depending on the one doing (or receiving) the messages, unsettling. The rules will change with the couple and the situation, and are not necessarily male or female specific.

Moreover, as old workplace hierarchies crumble or shift and women increasingly occupy senior positions, other intimacies such as touching, shaking hands, embracing or hugging have become a female initiated enterprise. At this stage, a wise position for men to take is to allow women to be the initiators and to look for responsible cues. Watch for signals and respond in kind with an appropriate hug, handshake, or cheek-kiss, nod or nothing. Australian larrikin humour has no place here.

This is probably one of the fall-outs of the #MeToo movement. Well-intentioned men are paying the price for bad behaviour of a few ignorant, unaware or unprincipled ones. The price is we are giving up the chance to be more spontaneous, unselfconscious and friendly. Being overly familiar now has inherent risk, perhaps a loss for both genders.

On the other hand, in a close-knit family unit, or even in a courting relationship, these acts of chivalry and intimacy would be seen more as a respectful and caring gesture – caritas in the Catholic lexicon – and probably treasured. I venture that any woman in this family, close or extended, would consider these acts to convey a strong message of esteem. Very clearly, a young mother will be appreciative for the shared (physical) strength and support of her male partner in all facets of home-building and raising children. A recent study found that some of the defining qualities which women find attractive in a man are unselfishness, confidence, aspiration and a degree of chivalry. Such a simple gesture as walking on the outside nearest the kerb to protect his partner from spray sent from a buggy (or car), are most likely taken as a mark of respect and caring.

Similarly, I suspect the corporate woman would acknowledge the reality that men are physically stronger than women. She would appreciate, and not reject, a trusted man's suggestion he escort her through a park at night or to a darkened car park – no obligation or expectations attached.

Until we assume responsibility for our behaviours towards women, whether it is her inspiration as a muse or to regain control over a feminine power they can't control, men remain exiled from what it means to truly understand the power of manhood, particularly related to the power of womanhood.

How do males find what it means to be a man? How do we achieve this behaviour change? Is one answer, for men and women, to know when to be a responsible and considerate person rather than just a male or a female? (Or other gender?)

Before we discuss this, I want to acknowledge the great behavioural changes that have happened already over the last generation or so.

A great deal has been already accepted by the younger generations. The younger generations are approaching manhood in a culture that is lurching towards a gender-neutral society. One that has moved so far from anatomy-based definitions of men and women, to one that recognises a person's self-assigned gender identity, regardless of the sex ticked on a birth certificate. Cultural, social, biological and political aspects have been completely redefined in terms of gender to a degree unimaginable a decade ago, certainly a generation ago.

The reality is, sex determination exists on a spectrum with genitals, chromosomes, gonads and hormones all playing a role, together with conditioning. Most fit into the male or female category, but about one in a hundred may fall in between.

The June 2021 issue of the *Journal of Paediatrics* reported a study by Dr Kacie Kidd that found that 9.2 per cent of high school students in the Pittsburgh school district consider themselves gender-diverse in some way.

A recent survey of a thousand millennials (those born between 1981 and 2000) found that half of them think gender is on a spectrum. At last count, there were at least some self-selective 50 loci along a spectrum between the poles of male and female. These include agender (no gender identity), gender fluid (gender identity shifts between male and female), LGBTIQ+ (lesbian, gay, bisexual, transgender, intersex, queer, plus). Transgender relates to a person whose sense of personal identity and gender does not match their biologic sex assigned at birth.

Based on these findings we need to recognise that men are not necessarily a homogenous group and that a range of activities should be tailored to meet the differing health needs of specific groups of men, particularly those where social disadvantage is most prominent. We need to acknowledge there is a considerable gender variation between men.

James Smith reported in the *Health Promotion Journal of Australia* (2007:18(1)), that practitioners, researchers and policymakers should consider it important to acknowledge the inequities faced by marginalised groups of men. For instance, a gay man, father, older man, young man, or Aboriginal man may face similar social, economic, cultural and political inequities as women, and different from each other. Simply, there are many different masculinities.

Clearly not all men enact hegemonic masculine behaviours. As a starting point, it has been acknowledged that the perpetuation of masculine dominant trait stereotypes during health encounters is unproductive. Such stereotypical expressions include "men are better able to cope with pain", or "men should be brave".

These need to be avoided. It becomes important to know the demographic you are trying to target. Recognising that stereotype hegemonic masculinity is being challenged through alternative forms of gender presentation is a critical step in moving men's health promotion forward. This requires an appreciation of how culture, sexuality, age, race, ethnicity and working class influence the multitude of masculine behaviours enacted by men.

So, biology need not be destiny, for men or women. And, gratefully, in these modern times there are few grotesque rituals or painful and embarrassing initiation ceremonies, ones which young men have to endure to gain peer acceptance and to mark the transition from boy to man.

This has made it difficult, but in reality, not necessary, to rely on the traditional roles of men and women for an idea of what it means to be a man. With gender equity now very much a real force, gender stereotypes have been turned inside out, or repudiated. We now have a society where we give equal status to female scientists, doctors and police or male nurses or male airline stewards, something rarely heard of thirty years ago. Fathers now stay at home looking after babies while the mother becomes the prime provider. Housework is shared with fathers doing their own ironing, cleaning and helping with the cooking. In this regard, men are often liberated when they find they can be very creative in the kitchen.

This shift should not be too surprising. New anthropological research offers an intriguing answer. *Work* by Lee T Gettler (January 2021 in *Scientists' Alliance*) suggests that nurturing fatherhood was embedded in male biology long before our ancestors became hunters and likely laid evolutionary foundations for our fathering roles. Caring fatherhood is not only core to men's parenting, but it may have come first in human evolution, before fathers developed strength to hunt large animals and provide food for their offspring.

Men's specialisation as hunters is generally possible only with the nutritional assurance provided by women's more consistent foraging of plants, insects and other small animals. Before this happened, low-cost behaviours such as food sharing and nurturing by fathers would have been a natural role for them, requiring a history of co-operation, trust and reliability. This would also give the male a better chance of mating, laying the foundations for trust. So, it is possible the caring father predated the provisioning father, rather than vice-versa.

This sits well with research which shows modern men who create in the kitchen alongside their partner increase their chances of mating, to have sex. Which, of course, may also have more to do with creating trust and friendships, as much as a prehistory legacy.

The Australian Institute of Family Studies report one-third of fathers now work flexible hours, and they are more involved in caring for their children, but their number of work hours usually do not change once a baby is born. More telling, only four per cent of fathers stay at home full time to look after their children. Compare this with Finland. Starting in 2021, all parents there have leave, regardless of their gender or whether they are the child's biological parents. Under the new law, each parent will be allowed to take 164 days off, or about seven months.

In Australia, we have a way to go. However, we acknowledge fathers are embracing precious time with their newborns as more workplaces move to offer equal paid parental leave for men and women. Leading the way is Deloitte Australia which now offers all new parents eighteen weeks of paid leave, as do a number of other large organisations. Compare this to my era in the sixties and seventies when fathers were not even allowed to watch the birth, let alone be encouraged to help with the baby. A great shame, in retrospect, as men were excluded from their children during a critical bonding period.

My own daughter's birth, in 1968, saw me acquire the mantle of being the first father in Queensland to witness their child's birth in hospital. Until then, ward matrons were adamant no father could attend births. There were concerns men would pass out during the procedure! When I approached my wife's obstetrician, an associate from rugby connections and asked if I could attend, he was doubtful. He gave me a letter of admission to give to the matron on duty as he couldn't overrule her in the ward.

As it turned out, she did let me in and, during the early stages, just before the birth, I was able as a physio to assist my wife with her breathing, etc. However, the matron insisted I go outside at the actual birth – in case I fainted. I was ushered outside for a couple of minutes and then invited back in, a marvellous bonding experience.

By the time my son was born two years later it was normal procedure to allow fathers in for the birth – a vote for common sense.

As men recede from their ivory towers, it is likely this feather of denial becomes ruffled as the vulnerability is revealed. However, as the feather is reshaped, the rewards involved in the transmission, for either or any gender, can be immense.

CHAPTER EIGHT

The Catastrophic Feather – Find the Power Within

'The difference between impossible and possible is simply a "degree of will". We all have strategies to prepare ourselves for a potentially stressful challenge, be it a sporting event, delivering a lecture or attending a corporate meeting. We may recite certain mantras or positively rehearse in our mind's eye the way we are going to play it. My special incantation was to recite (or sing, or listen to) the words from *Carmen Jones*, a film adaptation of Bizet's opera *Carmen*. It was the aria sung by the boxer Husky, *Stand up and fight*.

> Stand up and fight until you hear the bell,
> Stand toe to toe, trade blow for blow,
> Keep punching till you make your punches tell,
> Show that crowd what you know,
> Until you hear that bell,
> That final bell,
> Stand up and fight like hell.

I called on these tactics before I climbed into a boxing ring or competed in a high-level game of football. I had great confidence the incantation made it possible to find a deeper strength. There is a power deep within which arises from the requirements humans have for survival, and encourages actions to meet those needs. It can be cultivated to accept changes and overcome fear, and involves having a sense of our own capacity and self-worth.

To quote Mike Tyson, 'Everybody has a plan until they get hit in the mouth.'

So, when mantras and positive thinking strategies are not enough, it is possible to tap into a reservoir of power within. This is a beautiful feather, one which every peacock should strive to attain. I had my first experience of it when I was forty years old. In 1983, I was attempting a pilgrimage to climb over the jungle clad cliffs of the notorious Kokoda Trail in the Owen Stanley Ranges of New Guinea. This was the scene of a bitter six-month battle in 1942 in which Australians were pitted against an overwhelming and unbeaten Japanese juggernaut.

As a young boy I always knew my father had been a soldier, and when asked about it he briskly passed it off. In those early years, I considered him as a rather aloof but solid background figure, not prone to extravagant displays of emotion or affection. He never presented the need for affirmations or touching, yet I had no doubt his life centred on our family.

On Anzac Day, he marched with his brother-in-law, then later, with his friends at the RSL Club. The mask slipped as the alcohol washed away some of his reserve. The men often laughed uninhibitedly at some incident of long ago, then talk in hushed respectful tones when remembering "poor old Fred", who "copped it", "over there". More mystery! It was a world I could not understand – a conspiracy of silence in their own inclusive camaraderie.

Chapter Eight The Catastrophic Feather – Find the Power Within

Some years later, my father died, suddenly and quite young. I remember my feelings of helplessness and shock when I found the Repatriation Commission attributed his death to attrition incurred on the Kokoda Trail. My shock was complete – he had taken his secret with him.

In 1983, I had a chance to act as medic for fifteen of Queensland's top army and air force cadets to walk the trail. (The veterans who fought there called it the "Kokoda Track", but it is officially called the "Kokoda Trail"). At this stage, almost no one attempted the odyssey, the actual battle was almost lost in history. After two hours of climbing carrying a twenty-five-kilo pack in 35 degrees Celsius and ninety per cent humidity and after leaving an Australian winter, I suddenly understood a little of what my father had been through.

Even though physically fit, I was devastated to realise that the struggle might be too much for me. I had boxed for the state and competed at tough club rugby and athletics, but nothing in my life had prepared me for this extent of adversity. I was quite ready to turn around there and then. I struggled around behind a large boulder and found myself sobbing loudly, gasping for air and calling on the ghosts of Kokoda for help. I channelled men who had been there before me and had been tested, like Corporal John Metson who was wounded in both ankles at the Battle of Isurava, and refused to let his mates carry him. Instead, he wrapped his hands and knees in rags and crawled for three weeks through the jungle. I called on other men I had read about who had struggled here, Bruce Kingsbury VC, Stan Bisset and his brother Butch. I called for my father.

Then, almost imperceptibly gently, hard against the rising tide of panic and impending failure, a quiet voice deep inside took command and ordered me to take stock – to be calm. I followed the order and responded by pushing myself, one step at a time, at my own pace, into the realm of mind over matter.

Many times, as the trek developed into an emotional roller-coaster, my new commitment and resolve forced me to confront myself. I was aware that my inhibitions were being peeled away, layer after layer revealing a clearer image of myself, a core devoid of trappings. It took us ten days to traverse the track, and the experience changed me profoundly. It served as a vehicle for inner discovery and transformation.

This revelation concerning the Kokoda Track and my dad's reticence to share with me, satisfied me for some years. But I still felt the full secret eluded me. That secret would be revealed from another, completely different, direction. In 1992, as a classical sculptor, I was asked to create a statue to commemorate the fiftieth anniversary of the Kokoda Campaign.

When I unveiled the statue at the anniversary event some of the men confided in me about private incidents during the campaign. By the time I got home that evening, I was very excited. It dawned on me that I had at last began to uncover the mystery that had teased and eluded me most of my life. I realised here was a story of magnitude and richness that had not been recorded. I would write a book – *The Silent Men*.

As I wrote their story I realised with a degree of fascination I had found a generation of forgotten, silent men. Psychologists have long reported that those who have suffered the atrocities of war find it difficult to communicate their experiences to anybody who has not encountered something similar.

Chapter Eight   The Catastrophic Feather – Find the Power Within

I was reminded of some lines penned by Sebastian Faulks in his novel *Birdsong*, a story of grim horrors of trench warfare in the First World War. The lines come from a soldier writing an introspective letter to his loved one after several months of witnessing and experiencing inhuman events:

> No child or future generation will ever know what this was like.
> They will never understand.
> When it is over, we will go quietly among the living and we will not tell them.
> We will talk and sleep and go about our business, like human beings.
> We will seal what we have seen in the silence of our hearts and no words will reach us.

The Department of Veterans Affairs' counselling service reports that seventy-five per cent of Second World War veterans suffered symptoms of what was then called "anxiety neurosis". Unknown to me, my father had been receiving psychiatric counselling and medication since the war.

By the time Australian troops returned from the tragedy of the Vietnam War, the condition was more clearly recognised and better diagnosed as post-traumatic stress disorder (PTSD). It has been brought into sharp focus more recently as the condition also affected troops arriving home from the Middle East Area Operation (MEAO), Iraq and Afghanistan conflicts.

Through these men, I have come to know my father. I have come to know the great burden that was placed on the shoulders of his generation, The Great Generation, as they are now known, and who carried the legacies of war all of their lives. Many of these men were already carrying legacies from their fathers who had fought in the First World War. Many of these men, their fathers, were diagnosed as suffering the effects of shell shock and were not adequately treated.

Their male-hood was overwhelmed with horrendous experiences which made it difficult for them to process, calibrate and share their emotions. They inherited the legacy which males historically accepted as their roles: the killing, the sacrifices, the loss, the guilt, the heroism, courage and love. It was not only the men who carried the burden. Wives played an active and supportive role in what for many were difficult years.

For them, the fears started the minute their husbands walked out of the door to go off to fight. Often, they wouldn't hear from them for weeks or even months. One of the hardest times for the women was the waiting for the arrival of the daily newspaper in order to look at the casualty lists, hoping they wouldn't see any names they knew. Most of my generation felt the reverberations of their struggles, and their losses. The hope was that we could put the ghosts behind us as we tried to gain a new definition of manhood. But it has been slow.

This experience prepared me for that greater shock of the threat to my mortality from the prostate cancer diagnosis at the age of fifty-two.

At the time, such was the neglected state of awareness of men's health issues, I didn't even know what my prostate was, or what it did. For the previous twenty years as a health professional, I had followed a disciplined lifestyle of exercise, diet and meditation, one which the gurus had promised would significantly lessen the risk of cardiac disease and cancer. Not completely true, I naively found.

To add to the shock, virtually any invasive treatment I could undertake had the potential of being nasty. At the time, surgery (radical prostatectomy) seemed to offer the best chance of survival. The predominant medical prognosis suggested that without treatment, I may have only three to five years to live. (The survival rate at five years post diagnosis was about sixty per cent; now it is 95.5 per cent). However, after surgery, there was a vicious trade off. I was left severely incontinent. This had a serious impact on my lifestyle, as well as my professional career, emotional health, exercise activity, sex life and relationships.

I was also suffering from erectile dysfunction, a situation I was not coping with. I became very despondent and developed reactive depression. Worse still, I could find no other man who had been through this process. I felt very isolated. In my mind, I was the only man in the world in this situation. My emotions became extremely raw, leading to a catastrophic reaction.

The frustration, anger – and, indeed, often rage –led me to resolve to change things. The alternative was to accept a seriously reduced lifestyle. Suicide appeared an attractive proposition. The vulnerable time was driving home from work, tired and devastated that love making may never be a reality again. I really was feeling hopeless and despairing.

It was then that my quiet entity, my silent voice, deep inside, took command again. The voice reminded me that some of my female physiotherapy colleagues treated women with incontinence. In desperation, I sought them out. They taught me how to execute standard pelvic floor muscle exercises, which I performed aggressively and with enormous motivation. The action began to improve the situation tremendously. While this was more acceptable and manageable in terms of my lifestyle, even if I leaked a little, I still found I was caught in a cycle of depression, one of the now obvious psycho-social legacies resulting from my choice of treatment.

I put an advertisement in the local paper seeking to meet any men who may have been diagnosed with prostate cancer and having similar side effects. Seventy men and their partners turned up at the meeting. From this meeting we formed the first prostate cancer support group in Queensland. With the help and resources of psychologist Susanne Chambers, we based our headquarters at the Cancer Council Queensland rooms.

From this, I hoped to find some answers to assist both me and the many other fellow sufferers I had so quickly found. We formed a core group of about a dozen men and their partners and I morphed into the role of unofficial convenor. We self-directed ourselves, developing three main aims: to support and educate ourselves, to create community awareness of prostate cancer and to encourage research into all aspects of prostate cancer. At this stage, I could not find one article of research in Australia on any aspect of prostate cancer.

I began engaging with several other emerging groups around Australia and was part of the excitement in 1999 when we consolidated as the Prostate Cancer Foundation of Australia, the now peak consumer body for prostate cancer in Australia. From there, we never looked back. No man needed to be alone again.

Our Brisbane group grew to be one of the largest in Australia, hosting 1000 members and there are now 170 groups nationally.

The next challenge was to improve my incontinence to another level. Some four years after diagnosis, I was awarded a Cancer Council Queensland travelling fellowship to study for six weeks at major hospitals dealing with prostate cancer in the United States. From this, I designed an intensive exercise program aiming to develop a highly efficient neuromuscular and vascular system which controls and supplies all the structures that form the pelvic and abdominal cavities. This meant endurance type training, running, cycling and resistance training, while integrating pelvic floor muscle activity.

After six months of this program, it virtually cured the problem. But the best result was that this also broke the depression cycle. In 2003 I published the full program in a book *Conquering Incontinence*, the first of its kind anywhere. It is still recommended reading in all support groups.

In the meantime, I had learned to satisfactorily rehabilitate and cope with my erectile dysfunction; there are many modern techniques for this now.

A particular challenge for men coming to terms with the diagnosis and treatment for prostate cancer was to confront and understand the process of grief and loss. We need to know of the four main stages of grief – denial, anger, depression and acceptance. That way, we can learn to accept the losses and embrace the new reality of our life. With acceptance, we gain three gifts – insight, compassion and wisdom. Adjustment often requires time and re-evaluation of what it means to be human; to be a male. (More on grief and loss in Chapter 10).

As Sam Keen has stated, 'This means going on a quest to rediscover the sacred fire that ignites in our belly. It may challenge our belief systems and values, one's faith and the purpose of being.'

There is no stipulated age group for the need for this quest to occur, but my experience has suggested it tends to occur more in the middle-age group as life's pressures impact. The next chapter explores this vulnerable age group.

CHAPTER NINE

The Burgeoning Feather – The Awakening and the Mid-Life Crisis

In the words of Confucius: 'We have two lives, and the second begins when we realise we only have one.'

When I was in my early forties, I was impressed with a *60 Minutes* TV program which posed several questions to male viewers: have you recently bought a new red sports car, climbed a mountain, written a book, had an affair? Incredibly, I ticked three out of the four. I had indeed recently bought a new red sports car; I had struggled over the Kokoda Trail and had written two books on sport injuries.

So, what was going on? The narrator of the program suggested such men may be going through a mid-life crisis. There could be as many reasons for this as there were men, however a few points seemed to be consistent.

Basically, there was an overarching feeling that they may be questioning everything they had devoted their lives to for the last couple of decades. They may be confused with their direction and self-purpose. There was an awakening – a burgeoning awareness that their lives were running on autopilot with no real goal in sight. Everything they had established felt stagnant, even stifling.

All it takes is an epiphany to cause one to realise that life is short and tomorrow is not promised. There is a strong consideration to walk away from a career deemed successful by society in an effort to pursue passion. Overall, there is a fear of running out of time. a feeling of being overwhelmed by the time left to fulfil one's dreams, prompting out-of-character decisions to take risks – such as buying a new car or climbing mountains.

A certain percentage of these men will also have the added responsibility of caring for ageing parents and adult offspring. As well, they will probably be dealing with mortgages and school fees, and a demanding career which has compromised their lifestyle concerning fitness and diet. Or conversely, their adult children may have recently left home, leaving them feeling adrift, creating a loss concerning the gradual withdrawal of their parenting role. Others may be experiencing a profound loss of something that has contributed to their identity until now. Bereavement, divorce, bankruptcy, redundancy or it may be more subtle such as a loss of youth and looks, or loss of lover or partner. Or, it may simply be a shifting of values. Values set when twenty may be significantly different now at fifty.

Another factor that has recently been found to particularly impact on middle-aged males is loneliness combined with social isolation. Research has revealed one in four Australian men aged 35-49 are very lonely, and one in six of all Australian men are very lonely.

Loneliness does not affect only one particular age group. Surprisingly, young people aged 18-25 have high rates of loneliness, despite being a group that appears to be well-connected through school and technology. We have known for twenty years that Australian males are lonelier than females. Loneliness is now a real health problem. As reported in the June 2023 issue of *The Male*, which highlights understanding loneliness, while data in this area is relatively new, especially in Australia, some of the established stats are extremely concerning. In terms of longevity, loneliness has the same rate of impact as smoking up to fifteen cigarettes a day, and it increases the likelihood of early death by 26 per cent, which is greater than the risk for obesity. Unchecked, loneliness has the potential to be one of the critical health issues of our time and it appears we all (scientists, health professionals and the public in general) are only now realising how big a deal it really is.

Like any health issue, being aware of it is the first step. Do a self-audit on how you are doing in terms of your meaningful relationships. It may be useful to join a support group or club, from bonsai to budgies – they are out there – hobbies, men's sheds, health support groups, volunteer at a local sporting club. (Chapter 17).

As an example, let me introduce you to a patient and friend of mine. Rob was at the top of his game. He appeared to have it all: successful law firm, business and golf clubs, showpiece house, the Ferrari, investment home unit, attractive and smart wife and an achieving family at prestigious schools. He was fit, healthy and had political ambitions and was well-connected. Then one morning, sitting at the bench press machine, digging deep for more power, he suddenly and unexpectedly burst into uncontrollable floods of tears, something he had not done since he was a child. Until recently, that is, when his father had died; a man he acknowledged had unerringly chartered Rob's life and career. His father's death brought the shock of realising that his life until now may have been on autopilot, controlled by others. He was particularly shocked by his lack of insight into the repressed nether world of his emotions, dreams and unrealised desires. Since that event, he had been steadily gaining the notion that he had allowed himself to be directed along the wrong path.

As a solicitor, he was questioning if his perspective of his career still upheld the honourable traditions of the law, principals he had studied many years ago. Was he working for justice, or was he using his profession only to create obscene wealth and ego-driven status?

At the same time, he was also confronted with the terror of his own mortality and the concept of an afterlife, a dark abyss which forced him to think of the purposefulness of his own life. He was reaching an epiphany that his own life may be a sham, hollow and meaningless.

As mentioned earlier, there are many ways to reach this pivotal axis; a life-threatening disease, a financial loss, an unexpected family breakdown, physical or mental burn out, a time when you begin to question everything about the pathway you have been dutifully treading. This phenomenon is often called mid-life crisis, an emotionally uncomfortable period that is a time to question priorities and adjust one's thinking, attitudes and beliefs to fit better with emerging emotional needs. It is a time of asking deep, probing questions. The old model is being challenged and ready for a makeover.

This is the same reaction I had when I was thrust into confronting my own mortality when diagnosed with prostate cancer. I asked the same probing questions and challenged my whole life's belief systems.

This was the appropriate feather, the burgeoning, the awakening feather, the one I could add to my increasingly striking display. Not all men are equipped to, or do, ask these questions which are self-actualisation in nature, or even think of asking them. Such moves generally occur in individuals who are insightful and can afford the time to ask, to ponder. Many may not be in this category and may not seek this enlightenment. These men can often become lost, defensive souls, going for a different image – the sports car, younger partners, motor bikes, climbing mountains.

But for another man, he is ready to go on a quest, an almost holy grail, as in the earlier quote from Sam Keen, to find what really ignites the fire in his belly. He will need to learn more about himself, become his own authority on himself and in the process rethink and seek his own definition of life's purpose. The journey will take time, maybe years, and there will be dark periods during this process.

As the quotation attributed to Confucius at the beginning of this chapter attests, when you understand that you only live once, then can you be truly free and living, for the second part of your life. Rob eventually quit law and became a successful interior designer.

To venture on this odyssey is simply a matter of asking questions. Some universal questions a man may need to ask:

- Who am I, and what place have I in the universe?
- Does my life, or any life, have a meaning?
- What am I striving for? The answer may be haunted by the quotation from Epicurius (341 BC) that 'Nothing is enough for the man for whom enough is too little.'
- What really drives me?
- What was/is my relationship with my father? And what influence did he project, negative and positive, on my life?
- And my mother? And family?
- And my wife? How do I relate to her? Do I regard her as

a chattel, a trophy wife, an asset to be wheeled out for impression? Do I treat her with respect? As an equal?
- Do I present as a patriarchal "puffer fish"? A pompous overstuffed authority who says, 'Don't you worry your pretty head over this. I will make the decision.' Specialists in all professions tend to do this well.
- What skills do I have that may be repressed? Creative? Work? Human?
- Have I suppressed an artist inside, trying to get out?
- What vocation really suits me best?
- What are my values? My standards? And who/what has set them?
- What would I fight for? And be willing to die for? Is war necessary? Would I try the antidote to warfare, Socratic dialogue, a situation where conflicts can be resolved by intellectual wrestling? Or would I beat my chest and rattle my sabre?
- What are my belief systems? Theist, or not?
- Is there evidence of a transcendent God or afterlife?
- What does it mean to be a male?
- Why do we have an opposite gender?
- What is the source of my self-esteem?
- How important is my sex drive? Does it define me?
- Why do I have a sex drive?
- Where do I sit on the gender spectrum?

The task for any individual who wants to be free is to fearlessly delve into and unshackle the authorities and myths that have unconsciously shaped and informed his life.

Educating young boys is a good start; more on this later. Challenging all previous roles placed on him by his institutions, school, churches, government, parents and history, will allow him to rebuild his identity from scratch. Let him begin to see life with greater insight and awareness, which may translate to living a fuller life with more complexity, more than the simple directives of the three Ps – procreate, protect and provide. These men have to be prepared to go through a process of change, which means entering a period of introspection and reinvention.

Elements of this reaffirmation may appear brutal, even cataclysmic, involving terrific upheaval, particularly when reconsidering career choices. Currently, people are predicted to change their careers up to five times, so men will be well advised not to fall into any job because they have been told to just "make a living", or because it offers security. It will be better to find and work towards a career which gives you a sense of significance, of meaning. This is done by releasing the unique individual inside; create something of lasting value, a healthier food, a smarter running shoe, a tractor, a better computer program, write a book.

He may need to expand himself and his context. Along with considering his career choice, he may need to be prepared to physically explore the world, experience new cultures, and move out of his comfort zone. He may be advised to not sacrifice wide-ranging curiosity and fascination for the world at large for small compartmental thinking. He may be advised to be involved with what is real, and often challenging. The journey is the important part, not the end. Note again Kahlil Gibran's quote at the beginning of the introduction. It alludes to the concept that you will not make changes in your behaviour until you challenge yourself. Without an opportunity to cope with adversity, your life will always be on autopilot, following someone else's script. You may need to find situations where you can remove veneers and trappings. You can climb a real mountain if you like, but it is not necessary; it can be a metaphorical one. Starting a new job, learning a new skill, writing a book, studying for a PhD. Befriend someone from a different culture, age group or interest group.

Unless you try to go where you haven't been before, unless you run the risk of falling into hidden crevasses and chasms, or hitting walls, unless you have to search for your inner strength, you will not reveal the true character or intellectual entity inside. It is worthwhile turning to ancient Greece here to consider Socrates. He states, 'Know thyself first.' (From the Delphic Maxims). This saying at the frontispiece of the Temple of Apollo at Delphi would challenge visitors first. This is reinforced by his (Socrates) famous dictum, 'The unexamined life is not worth living.' During this process, you will shed many coats and recalibrate who you are, or who you think you are.

There is a word of caution here. The life sciences challenge the assumption that we may have an inner core, or a single voice. They contend that humans are organisms, which we are, and organisms are algorithms and not individuals. That is, humans are an assemblage of many different algorithms lacking an inner voice or a single self. An external algorithm may know me much better than I can ever know myself.

Further, Dr Fiona Kerr, an Australian neuroscientist, reports that people of all ages have admitted to her that they distract themselves from this process. That is, they deliberately practice "busyness", because they don't want to reflect. People often resist the idea of an inward journey for fear they might not like what they find.

The writer Yuval Harari has emphasised that, in this modern era it may not be that easy to identify our authentic will, or even desirable. When we try to listen to ourselves, we are often flooded by a cacophony of conflicting noises. We sometimes don't want to hear our authentic voice because it might disclose unwelcome secrets, desires, addictions and behaviours, genetic or brainwashed, and make uncomfortable requests. Many people take great care not to probe themselves too deeply. Human dramas unfold when people have uncomfortable desires. Modern technology, biochemistry, dataism and artificial intelligence threaten to hijack and change our idea of "examined life". It will soon be possible for technologies to gain control and redesign our will. It foresees a world that does not revolve around the desires and experiences of any humanlike beings. Once technology enables us to engineer bodies, brains and minds, we can no longer be certain about anything. The human body itself might undergo an unprecedented revolution thanks to bioengineering and direct brain to computer interfaces. We must be prepared for this unstoppable event. We will need to reinvent ourselves again and again.

So, should you trust yourself? As the oldest advice in the book says, 'Know thyself.' This advice is becoming even more urgent. As Yuval Harari further warns us, we now have serious competition, Amazon, Google, Coca-Cola and the government are all racing to hack you. Not your smartphone, not your computer, not your bank account – they are in a race to hack you and your organic operating system.

With the help of algorithms, companies can inject content

straight into consumers' everyday lives. They prioritise the content that we consume including what we see, when we see it, how prominent it is and how long we see it for. They influence a third of our decisions on major shopping sites such as Amazon.

The algorithms are watching you right now. Whether it's Siri or Alexa, they are listening to your questions and finding out what your interests are, where you go, what you buy, who you meet, your heartbeat, your health. They influence what and where you buy and what you like. Once they get to know you better than you know yourself, they could control and manipulate you. You will live in the matrix and authority will shift to them.

If you don't want to go along with this ride, and would like to retain some control of your life and your future, you have to run faster than the algorithms, get to know yourself before they do.

Men seeking change will have to examine the programs running in their hard drive that are not serving them: they may need to rewire the brain. The final destination may be vague, and may often change along the way. It may take many years; the quest may have to go back to the beginning, to the "big bang", to search for clues as to who we are, a speck in a vast cosmos. It may well be a lifelong learning experience as a phrase often misattributed to Michelangelo attests, when he was eighty-seven and wrote on one of his artworks, *ancora imparo* – 'I am still learning.' The quote is actually from Seneca's letter to Lucilius published in 65 AD during the last year of the author's life when he was almost seventy years old. It is a heartening revelation that life's experiences teach us that to stop learning is to stop creating. The search for knowledge should never end.

This will be a search for the drive which stirs an individual's innate passions and fulfils his deepest inner self, uncomplicated by any earlier influences. Simply, he will be searching for what developmental psychologists term "intrapersonal intelligence". The quest here is to have an advanced understanding of himself – think of this not as egotism, but of self-awareness.

All change involves a certain amount of loss, whether it be a search for awareness or a life-threatening disease. A particular challenge for men coming to terms with the impact of certain traumatic incidents, including the diagnosis and treatment of diseases and cancers, especially prostate cancer, the most common cancer facing men, is to confront and understand the process of grief and loss. The next chapter will help to understand this process.

CHAPTER TEN

The Grieving Feather

*'True happiness comes only from a life of meaning
– of doing what was worth doing,'*
– Aristotle

Any life-threatening disease, be it cardiac, diabetes, liver or cancer, has the ability to profoundly alter the way we think of ourselves and our existence. Prostate cancer is the most commonly diagnosed cancer in Australia and the most commonly diagnosed among Australian men. As already stated, one out of six men and their families will confront this disease. When I was diagnosed with prostate cancer in 1996 I had absolutely no idea that my heroic spontaneous decision to surgically remove the prostate would create a lasting, disastrous impact. The decision was easy – slash, burn or poison (surgery, radiation, chemotherapy or hormone therapy.) I had witnessed my father endure a terrible death from bowel cancer and I wanted my cancer out as quickly as I could. But it wasn't straightforward. I experienced first-hand that prostate cancer treatment, or the disease itself, has the potential to produce great loss. To treat localised prostate cancer, either by surgical (prostatectomy – removal of the prostate) or radiotherapy intervention, raises the prospect of losing our lives, our careers and ability to work. Just as critically we may also lose control of certain bodily functions, in particular continence (urinary and faecal) and our erectile function, which can then impact on self-worth and relationships. Advanced/metastatic prostate cancer, where the cancer has escaped beyond the prostate, will encroach on a greater number of body functions.

As prostate cancer is driven by testosterone, the initial treatment of advanced or metastatic prostate cancer involves depriving the body of its main source of testosterone. This is achieved either by surgical castration (orchidectomy, surgically removing the testes) or chemical castration (ADT – androgen deprivation therapy, depriving the body of male hormones). Either way, the resultant testosterone loss will seriously impact on major functions in the body. I found out that one of the other consistent side-effects of all treatment may be erectile dysfunction (ED) which, together with a reduction of penile size, has the potential to penetrate to the core of what we perceive it means to be a male.

As the previous chapter discussed mid-life crises, this may be an appropriate place to have a further discourse on ED, a condition that can become obvious in your forties, and a certain possible trigger for setting off an "awakening".

ED is an inability to achieve and/or maintain an erection satisfactory for sexual intercourse. It is one of the leading causes of negative change in male behaviour. A recent paper from Australian researchers Suzanne Chambers and colleagues reviewed studies that have examined the role of masculinity in men's response to erectile problems and the effects on quality of life after prostate cancer treatments.

Many of the studies reported that erectile dysfunction affected men's sense of masculinity and this was often a course of anxiety or embarrassment that impacted on their wellbeing. For most men, masculinity is an important factor in their experience of prostate cancer treatment and should be a part of the discussion between men, their partners and the treatment team.

When struggling with erectile dysfunction very soon after treatment, I became aware that the psycho-social aspects following the diagnosis and treatment of prostate cancer, have the ability to dramatically affect your life, to change the way you view it and the way you live it. It soon became obvious that this aspect of the disease was one of the main reasons for men needing support and joining the support group.

This loss in identity can quickly propel a man through the various stages which accompany this loss. So it is important to know and seek assistance to understand the four main stages of grief-denial, anger, depression and eventually acceptance. This feather, the grieving feather, is surely the one we need to grasp, to understand and to embrace.

Men are extremely effective dealing with denial. With anything that challenges our perspective of who we believe we are there is a tendency to think, 'this isn't happening' – disease, ageing, mistakes of any sort. It is a defence mechanism to deal with the rush of overwhelming emotion.

However, as reality sets in, and we are faced with the pain of the loss, we are quick to anger, looking for somebody or something to blame – other people, a higher power, the universe or life in general. In my support group men, unequipped to deal with the losses, often lashed out blaming diet, not enough sex, too much sex, stress, any amount of unscientific conspiracy theories.

Sadness sets in as we begin to understand the loss and its effect on our life and we can pass into a stage of reactive depression. This may last days, weeks or months, until finally with insight and perhaps support, we can move on to acceptance, acknowledging the reality of the loss. The situation can't be changed. Although there will be a degree of sadness, it is now possible to start moving forward with life. As erectile dysfunction was one of the main side-effects which I found led to grieving in our group, it is worthwhile highlighting the disorder.

Erectile dysfunction is common in older men and is often linked to factors such as being overweight, arterial insufficiency, having diabetes (affecting up to four in every five men over the age of forty with diabetes), high blood pressure and high cholesterol, men who are living with depression and anxiety, or being a smoker. As well, in some cases, it has been found there is an increased risk of ED which may be passed on, or inherited, through our genes. A tiny variation in the DNA code which occurs very close to a gene called SIM1 has been implicated. The median age of a prostate cancer diagnosis is sixty-six, so some men may have already begun to experience some erectile problems as they age, even before a prostate cancer diagnosis. About forty per cent of men will experience an erectile problem at some time at the of age forty, fifty per cent at age fifty, sixty per cent at age sixty, and the numbers increase with age.

There is not much a man can do about ageing, but apart from age-related problems affecting his ability to maintain an erection, there can be a psychological component to consider. As men's health doctor Michael Gillman reports, this may include such things as relationship issues with either his partner or family (or both), stress, financial worries, fatigue, continence issues and medication for co-morbidities. A psychological component can quickly result in a cycle of sexual performance anxiety. So there is a need to look at physical and psychological aspects when addressing erection problems.

It was once usual (forty years ago) for a man to have a prostatectomy and then simply wait to see whether erections returned, which could be months, years or never. What is certain, then and now, is that if it did return, it would never be as good as it was. The delay could be caused by neurogenic, arthritogenic, venogenic or psychogenic issues (or a mixture of these), but the longer it takes to treat and revive erectile function, the more difficult it will be to achieve a satisfactory outcome. An unfortunate side-effect of this delay is that the lack of a regular blood supply to oxygenate penile tissues that occurs during an erection can cause scarring and fibrosis of the penis in extreme instances.

A treatment program for erectile dysfunction from any cause should involve a doctor with particular expertise in male sexual dysfunction. In addition to addressing causes from a number of medical conditions along with drug treatments, management options include using tablets known as PDE5 (phosphodiesterase type 5) inhibitors (Viagra, Cialis or Levitra). If one brand doesn't work, try another. If tablets don't stimulate a response, self-injection of prostaglandin E1 into the shaft of the penis is a frequently used option. Alprostadil (which is chemically identical to prostaglandin E1) is also available as an intraurethral injection to be employed as an aid for inducing an erection, Muse™. A third rehabilitation option is a vacuum pump, which draws venous blood into the penis rather than fresh arterial oxygenated blood, as with a normal erection. Once the blood is drawn into the penis, a tension ring is placed around the base of the penis, maintaining an erection.

When other methods to overcome erectile problems have failed and a couple still desire an intimate sexual relationship, an intra-cavernosal implant can be considered. This consists of two inflatable tubes surgically implanted within the penis, along with a fluid reservoir kept in the lower abdomen behind the pubic bone, and a pump located in the scrotum. Once installed, the implants are undetectable and have a good history of reliability and satisfaction.

It must be re-stated, however, it is critical to search for a cause of erectile dysfunction. As virtually any form of medical treatment for prostate cancer, as well as a range of other conditions, has the potential to compromise erections and libido, it is no wonder that, when this befalls a previously sexually active male, a prospective drama begins to unfold.

There will be an alarming realisation by the individual of a dampening of the whole delicious anticipatory cycle (diminished reactions to such things as perfume or the flash of a thigh), leading directly to a potentially negative impact on relationships. With prostate cancer, besides dealing with the initial trauma following the diagnosis, a man will quickly suffer a degree of pathos as he realises he may have lost, possibly forever, the central function by which he has previously defined himself as a male. This is a period when this loss could spiral him into thoughts of suicide. There is often regret for his choice of treatment.

This is when counselling and education are essential. The man will need to be reminded he is alive now because he chose to narrow the odds of dying from this disease. This trade-off looks like a large price to pay now but in the long run, it won't be. Over time most men will accept this compromise.

As the convenor of a prostate cancer support group for twenty years, I was privileged to share many cases involving erectile dysfunction. One concerned a man in his late seventies who advised us that when he was undergoing his own hormone deprivation treatment he endured many years without sex. He commented that even though it was tough, once you've adapted to the changes and reassessed your life you will find life can be pretty rich. His loss of libido wasn't a problem. He said if a pretty girl displayed an attractive décolletage, he would automatically look, and then laugh to himself. He had completely lost the desire to do anything about it, and it didn't bother him. He could live life very well without sex.

Then there was the Kokoda Trail veteran who, at eighty years, had been impotent for years and was about to get married to a much younger lady. He wanted to know how he could reignite his erection. He was advised to try a penile injection, which he did. He reported it worked perfectly. I last saw him when he was eighty-five and he said he could still use the injection. He unfortunately passed away at ninety, from a heart condition. Many men from the support group were still using the injection effectively after twenty-five years, with no obvious side-effects such as penile scarring.

A different perspective, as the first man revealed, is that there may be some who actually accept and welcome this sexual dysfunction. Just as some of us may need to learn that a woman is more than a support system for her vagina and breasts, men are more than their erectile ability.

Perhaps we can look at some words of wisdom from antiquity.

In Plato's *Republic*, a man of advanced years described the relief of no longer being obsessed with sex. Many of his fellows, he said, lived in their memories of the pleasures of youth. But not him. He now had time for creative and cerebral outlets.

Nor, apparently, was Sophocles concerned by the impact of advancing age. When the great dramatist was asked whether he still made love to women, he answered, 'Good heavens, no. I have gladly made my escape from that barbarous, savage monster.' (However, I suspect he may not have made this judgment if he was a younger man).

This sentiment is echoed by Cicero and Seneca as they cite various authorities: 'The most fatal curse given to mankind is sensual greed,' and 'Age frees us from youth's most dangerous failings.'

These sentiments cannot be taken lightly. One might expect such pronouncements from clerics and individuals who have voluntarily accepted poverty, chastity and obedience, but not from aristocratic geniuses who have tasted the best the ancient world had to offer.

Even though it is easy to suspect that these writings may be a rationalisation of a man making the best of a bad bargain, I believe there may be a message of liberation of sorts if a man can work through his loss into acceptance.

Gandhi stated that he could never accomplish what he wanted to do unless he could channel the energy which he would normally burn (waste) on his libido and sex drive. He added that if he could take that energy and direct it in the proper way, he could liberate India. Which he did.

There are other benefits to be derived from acceptance. Over time, psychologists suggest we may acquire three gifts – insight, compassion and wisdom.

This enlightenment has the potential to lead to another "gift" that a life-threatening condition can disclose, an emerging need to live a meaningful and contented life, as suggested by Aristotle at the beginning of this chapter. There is such a phenomenon as "post traumatic transformational growth". This concept holds that people who endure psychological struggle following adversity can often see positive growth afterward.

Not everyone experiences growth after trauma. Psychologists have found that there are certain traits that increase its likelihood, such as optimism, extroversion and openness to new experience. Supportive resources and clinical treatment can also facilitate progress, particularly when dealing with a fixed mindset versus a growth mindset.

I have had this experience myself after my own diagnosis of prostate cancer. After setting myself the same questions, as well as helping me to come to terms with my own situation, the best outcome was it helped me to redefine a satisfying and contented purpose for my existence.

Conquering this hypothetical mountain provides us with the capacity to gain new insights and wisdom, to cut through nonsense, sham, dogma and other people's expectations of who you are and how you define yourself. Not unlike climbing a real mountain, this introspective journey is not only a journey upwards. As you work towards acceptance, veneer is stripped away, like a chrysalis, revealing the purest butterfly. This journey doesn't change you; it reveals you; you were always there.

The idea is to learn to trust your inner voice and act on it. Allow me to expand this thought.

Someone has given you a magic tonic, and miraculously you can redesign your life. Imagine writing a book with you as the central character, the hero, achieving whatever you would like. You can rewrite your own mythology. This means you can be adventurous, asking such questions as, is there a more courageous, risk-taking or creative way to achieving the goals of your hero (you)? He must question his intentions and motivations. Should the hero ask more of himself? More than he has been given credit for by external and limiting authorities? Should he allow room to develop and search for a deeper strength? Your central character, you, must also have the audacity to dream big and not be afraid of failing. Shut out negative and confining barriers, set from outside. Filter out other systems of belief that have been infecting your soft drive, and the mythology that has been presented to you on your hard drive.

During this process, do not be frightened to be part of something larger than your own life – plan something that may last long after you've gone.

Another word of caution; seriously monitor Google, Amazon, super-intelligent machines and algorithms that can manipulate your emotions with uncanny precision. The voice we hear inside our heads can be twisted by marketing experts reflecting state propaganda, ideological brainwashing and commercial advertisements.

CHAPTER ELEVEN

The Manly Feather

'The good physician treats the disease:
The great physician treats the patient who has the disease,'
— **Sir William Osler.**

When I was blindly burgeoning through adolescence in the 1950s and 60s, there was no structured advice to becoming a man. Our generation learned by osmosis, mainly emulating and matching our "silent" fathers, men who mostly were returned service men. My teachers invariably were from the same mould. Many were still affected by their war experiences, were stoic, tough and demanded strong rituals and values inherited from Crusaders and Victorian military and theistic traditions.

Mothers taught us many skills, mainly humanistic – good manners, to be respectful, to be authentic, honest, to take responsibility for mistakes and how to manage stress.

There was nothing specifically written or taught on how to be a man, but I gorged on a feast of *Boy's Own Paper* and adventure books, generally reinforcing epic and daring sagas and military heroes. Such titles as *The Count of Monte Cristo*, *Moby Dick*, the various *Biggles* adventures, *The Last of the Mohicans*, *The Three Musketeers*, *Danger Patrol* and stories of mountaineering and the conquest of Everest.

So, I ask what could break the cycle that equates manhood with toughness and stoicism? And what can be done to develop a healthier attachment to women? Do we journey to women or away – or both? On the other side of the coin, this may not be just a male's problem. What can women do to break the cycle? (And, of course, women have well started).

Perhaps one of the most influential pieces of literature of the era which transcends these themes was written by the India-born British laureate poet Rudyard Kipling. His poem *If* is one of ultimate inspiration that tells us how to deal with different situations in life. The poet conveys his ideas about how to win this life and, above all, to be a good human being.

Kipling wrote the poem in 1896, as if giving advice to his son. The poem almost immediately was hailed as a magnificent tribute to many of humankind's greatest virtues – staying composed under stress, remaining humble when victorious, never despairing when defeated, and always retaining honour and authenticity.

I first read the poem as a schoolboy and there are times that it still inspires and comforts me. I consider it remains a valid protocol for any generation, of any gender. I include it here for starters.

>*If* by Rudyard Kipling
>If you can keep your head when all about you
>Are losing theirs and blaming it on you,
>If you can trust yourself when all men doubt you,
>But make allowance for their doubting too;
>If you can wait and not be tired by waiting,
>Or being lied about, don't deal in lies,
>Or being hated, don't give way to hating,

And yet don't look too good, nor talk too wise:
If you can dream – and not make dreams your master;
If you can think – and not make thoughts your aim;
If you can meet with Triumph and Disaster
And treat those two impostors just the same;
If you can bear to hear the truth you've spoken
Twisted by knaves to make a trap for fools,
Or watch the things you gave your life to, broken,
And stoop and build 'em up with worn-out tools:
If you can make one heap of all your winnings
And risk it on one turn of pitch-and-toss,
And lose, and start again at your beginnings
And never breathe a word about your loss;
If you can force your heart and nerve and sinew
To serve your turn long after they are gone,
And so, hold on when there is nothing in you
Except the Will which says to them: 'Hold on!'
If you can talk with crowds and keep your virtue,
Or walk with Kings – nor lose the common touch,
If neither foes nor loving friends can hurt you,
If all men count with you, but none too much;
If you can fill the unforgiving minute
With sixty seconds' worth of distance run,
Yours is the Earth and everything that's in it,
And – which is more – you'll be a Man, my son!

As my life progressed, my behaviour very much echoed the traditional model for the various stages of manhood, including how they relate to toughness. These are the essential and unambiguous changes that will occur, the developmental stages a man will pass through as he ages. These broad stages are generally earned and celebrated by rituals, allowing the boy/man to be accepted by his peers, the only ones who can truly acknowledge this status. These changes, triggered by hormones, will happen whether they are celebrated by a ritual or not. They are primitive and as I relate to them now (below) I have tried to superimpose them on modern influences.

Stage 1. 0-twenty years, the athletic or testosterone years. During this period, a boy will be testing himself to reveal what he is made of, to try to place himself at the top of the gene pool.

Here he is at his most competitive, and probably most aggressive, seeing who is the fastest, strongest and bravest, the most daring, doing what needs to be done to reach the top of the pecking order. This is the stage when some men may be endowed with hotness delusional syndrome (HDS) – a condition in which he would consider himself to be "the universal gift to women". Not all boys will be immersed in this. The quieter, sensitive and "nerdy" types develop their own way of presiding.

Ultimately, this frenzied and often confusing and challenging period is intended to present himself as an attractive proposition to a prospective partner or, in some societies, multiple partners. There is a robust debate that men are supposed to be polygamous and that no one is cut out for monogamy. Consider the challenges for monogamy when grappling with divorce, infidelity, arranged marriages and the welfare of children. From an evolutionary perspective, playing the field is a way to get diverse DNA into as many beds as possible. But history and experience suggest the rewards for monogamy mean we should aim for it. Researchers

(Fletcher et al, *Perspectives in Psychology*, 2015) conclude that romantic love is a "commitment device" for motivating pair-bonding, facilitating the massive investment required to rear children. This arrangement is also linked to enjoyment, security, better health and survival, and plays a critical role in our evolution.

Stage 2. twenty to forty years, the procreative and protective years, fuelled by the sex drive. At this stage, he has taken or not taken a partner(s) and is probably raising or not raising children. This is the stage where he assumes ownership, will attempt to become king of his castle and protect it and all those in it to the death. This is the period when he will resist projecting any signs of weakness or vulnerability. He is at his warrior-like best as he strives to protect and provide for his family.

Stage 3. forty to -forty-five years, the elders. To age gracefully, he must aspire to become a wise elder. By this stage his children generally have a degree of independence. The elders were more than just an asset to the tribe – they were essential. They were revered. Long before information, history and knowledge were encapsulated by writing, the elders were our only font of experience and good judgement. The younger men learned tribal skills by the sharing of wisdom and knowledge through storytelling, participation in hunting and field work and through the well-established practices of showing, telling and doing. They were the very foundation of continuity, stability and certainty for the tribe. In the larger scheme, an elder has achieved life's main purpose, to pass his genes on to ensure the survival of the species, to ensure the survival of life and to raise his children. Physically, he is now generally well past his use by date. Every anatomical structure, muscle, ligaments, cartilages and joints particularly, are significantly deteriorating and his strength, endurance and agility are starting to fade.

However, with his life experiences, he has hopefully gained wisdom and some "rat-cunning" (or not). As one of the elders, he can be part of the tribal council and assist in law-making, and the policies and business of maintaining a tribe. Until recently, there would be no women in this echelon. Unfortunately, there will be a cohort of men who fall into the "or not" category. Some may be endowed with the "grumpy old man" syndrome. They believe they have reached the end of relevance and may have become cynical, sarcastic and intolerant.

In recent decades, as our life span has increased and all age groups now have access to unlimited information at their fingertips, the elders' importance has been much diluted; age discrimination is unbridled. There is a tendency to view older people, particularly in the workplace, as more likely to be sick, slow-working and intolerant of new technology.

Researchers have found none of this to be true, particularly in respect of older people in management or leadership positions. The nation, institutions and companies are being deprived of a terrific resource, a wellspring of experience and wisdom. This is a stigma which needs to change. There should be no upper limit for retirement.

Stage 4. fifty-five years and beyond – final transition to old age, also called senescence, the final stage of the human life span. Old age is generally divided into three stages – young old (fifty-five to sixty-five years), the point when our DNA noticeably starts to degenerate; middle old (sixty-six to eighty-five), traditionally called elderly and begins at sixty-five in Australia, sixty-eight in Britain, sixty-nine in France, seventy in Italy and seventy-four in Spain;

and finally old old (eighty-five and older), when bones become brittle as they lose calcium and other minerals. Other changes occur in individual cells and whole organs, resulting in changes in function and appearance.

Gerontologists report that by age seventy seniors have at least three chronic diseases to deal with, such as deafness, blindness and arthritis etc. By eighty years, they can have seven comorbidities. Heart disease, stroke, cancer and diabetes are among the most common, causing two-thirds of deaths each year. This is also the main age group for falls and balance problems, delirium, dementia and depression.

Evidence from the 2006 English longitudinal study of ageing found that, on average quality of life for men actually increases from fifty years as they lose dependent children and move into retirement. Not quite so for women, who are often carers, were not as well educated and often did not have the same retirement benefits as males, particularly so for single females. For males, quality of life was found to peak at sixty-eight from where it gradually starts to decline.

For most males, even though there may be a quiet acknowledgement that life is finite, there is also a contrasting denial that this relates immediately to them. As Woody Allen has been quoted, 'I am not afraid of death, I just don't want to be there when it happens.'

Of all who have considered the subject, none perhaps has done it more significantly than Cicero, from whose observations on age I select a couple of compelling sentences.

'Fools impute (attribute) their frailties and guilt to old age,' he said. 'The fact is that the blame for all complaints of that kind are to be charged to character, not to a particular time of life: unreason and churlishness cause uneasiness at every time of life.'

And, 'Men who have no resources in themselves find every age burdensome. There is a quite pure and cultivated life which produces a calm and gentle old age.'

He adds, 'If they have adapted to the qualities of culture and active exercise of the virtues, and maintained this at every period, the harvest they produce is wonderful.'

There appears to be a recognisable portal one passes through when these men accept they are now facing their mortality – death is imminent. This is when they become aware that many body systems are breaking down and can't be effectively resurrected. It is a moment of reckoning, a chance for review and a realisation they should not waste time on unimportant issues. In many ways, it can be a liberation, an event that only tolerates truthfulness.

These thoughts are reflected by the architype Central European activist and writer Arthur Koestler, penned after his imprisonment by Franco and the Spaniards in 1937, and then by the French in a concentration camp at the outbreak of the Second World War.

'Most of us were not afraid of death, only the act of dying; and there were times when we overcame even this fear. At such moments, we were free men without shadows, dismissed from the ranks of the mortal; it was the most complete experience of freedom that can be granted a man.'

So maybe we cannot live until we assimilate the truth of our mortality. Until you learn to die, you don't know how to live. Preparing to die well is one of the most important things a human being must do as they age.

This is when most elders can enter the realm of the sage, although many will not.

Until this modern era, not many people lived to this stage – on average, fifty-five years. Because of a high child mortality rate, the life expectancy of a man in Egyptian Pharaoh's time (5000 years ago) was around thirty to forty years. However, with privilege, luck and good genes, it was possible to live much longer. Ramses II lived until ninety (1304 BC-1214 BC), but Tutankhamun was not so lucky; he died at nineteen (1343 BC-1323 BC). Even until the beginning of the nineteenth century, the life expectancy for European men was forty-five years and even younger for women.

In most primitive cultures, by sixty years the majority of men had a serious loss of physical abilities, but had reached the age where their insight and life-experiences gave them the opportunity to be elevated to the status of sage. A sage is one who has attained such a state of being that he accepts what cards the universe has dealt. His life becomes tranquil and there can be some mellowing to allow him to deal with ethereal matters. These men are generally above physical realities and have accepted the actualities of life. Their insights can be a calming influence on younger generations. I believe to grow old without accumulating wisdom and becoming a mentor is to strip the last half of life of its *raison d'être*.

However, having considered all of this, I must mention an exciting alternative and hopeful caveat. Until recently, our understanding of ageing was defined by the *Merck Manual of Geriatrics*, which called ageing an 'inevitable, irreversible decline in organ function that occurs over time even in the absence of injury, illness, environmental risks or poor lifestyle choices.'

However, in 2010, over two remarkable days, the Royal Society of London convened a conference on ageing. As stated in David Sinclair's 2021 edition of his book *Lifespan*, the biogerontologist David Gems concisely summarised the meeting.

He wrote that advances in our understanding of organismal senescence (ageing) are all leading to a momentous conclusion: that ageing is not an inevitable part of life but rather a 'disease process with a broad spectrum of pathological consequences.'

In this way of thinking, cancer, heart disease, Alzheimer's, arthritis, kidney disease, diabetes and all diseases which we commonly associate with ageing, are not necessarily diseases themselves, but symptoms of something greater.

Put more simply and perhaps even more seditiously, ageing itself is a disease and a risk factor.

The science world is beginning to unite in this new science of ageing which is the cause of most of our morbidities. They have committed to tackle them at their source – ageing, the disease. They consider this disease is treatable.

Collectively, they are looking at many avenues, from supplements to lifestyle. These range from supplementing compounds such as NMN (nicotinamide mononucleotide), which has already demonstrated abilities to extend lifespan, gene therapy, to eating fewer calories, epigenetic reprogramming, adding certain vitamins, to the value of appropriate exercise and meditation. Watch this space.

Considering all this, and as with all behavioural change, particular men may have to develop some insight as to what is acceptable. Admit there is a problem, particularly with the consequences of male dominance, then be prepared to change. To do this, he will need to spend time searching and learning what it means to become a man in this present era, and thus define his identity and purpose. He will need to learn where he fits in with all aspects of gender equity, including how it relates to the now outmoded three Ps. In this context, the feminist revolution has exposed how life has seriously discriminated against women. An unintended consequence of this tectonic shift has also crippled the male psyche. In this modern era, where there is a lack of meaningful manhood rituals, and not often a strong father figure, a boy may need to find these things himself. It may be important for him to learn the discipline and joy of solitude, to practise self-reflection.

To better understand his male-hood, to gain perspective on the forces of his testosterone and the influence of women, it may be a worthy experience to travel by himself. That might be to live in a flat in the city or suburbs, enter a college or university, move to the next city or overseas or leave the familiar influences which have formed him, the positive and negative.

What if he went on a journey? While away, living by his own wits, with either a mentor or by himself, he may search for and ask the correct questions, the new rites of passage, the ones which will take him to lucid manhood. It might reinforce these are things which are difficult to do by himself. A counsellor, online course or the correct resources will be helpful.

As part of the journey, he will need to learn more about womanhood and the basic behavioural differences between males and females.

In my first week at university, I learned some significant lessons and gained insights previously unknown to me. During anatomy dissection classes as one of the few males in a class of thirty-five females, I would share a cadaver at a table with five female students.

As we hovered over the body, dissecting and studying anatomy, I could carry out a one-on-one conversation with one of the young women (all aged eighteen, I was twenty). Then two others at the table would talk to each other, then the other two would also talk, but amazingly, I realised they were all listening to each other's conversations and taking part in them and responding when necessary. This multi-tasking competence absolutely surprised me. I realised then that women network quite differently to men.

Their conversation revolved around topics I wasn't used to: clothes, beauty, family, often including sick or elderly members (a nurturing aspect I would rarely discuss outside the family), their own health, social life and parties, sometimes about the cute medical student on the table next door. But never about sport or cars or things which interested me.

I was also rather surprised they weren't always attracted to the alpha male – the sports jock, the big man on campus. Most seemed to gravitate towards the witty, the humorous and the sensitive literary type.

Over the next three years, these women became my best friends. I became privy to conversations which were immediately inclusive and uniquely feminine, very removed from the predictable and guarded topics of my male friends. I quickly learned not to talk over them, or try to fix their problems. I realised one of the requirements for their friendship and trust was simply to listen to them. They didn't need me to solve their problems, as men often try to do; they mainly needed respect and acknowledgment.

Importantly, I never delivered any romantic cues to any of them, preferring to keep my relationship with them as "one of the girls", a status they jokingly granted me and I graciously accepted.

I never complemented them or commented on their looks, bodies, accessories or clothes, which was challenging as they were an attractive group.

They appreciated there was no other agenda when I potentially revealed my male vulnerability and asked for assistance with my weaker subjects, physics, neurology or pathology. The only time it was acknowledged I may have been really helpful to them was during biology classes when it was essential to pith a frog. This was a method of killing a frog by inserting a large probe into the frog's neck, severing the spinal cord. I remember pithing ten at one class. Perhaps I was channelling my hunter-gatherer ancestors or maybe I was conditioned to dispassionately deal with life and death by my early farm upbringing. There was definitely a combined feminine reluctance to do this.

I must confess my other asset as a male among my female colleagues, was my ability to act as a conduit for introductions. This was still an era where it was considered very forward and generally improper for women to make advances to males. I still fostered and mixed with many male friends from other faculties and from sport connections. I played club rugby, competed at athletics and still boxed (without hitting anyone), and knew a great deal of athletes and medical students. I was very useful to them here.

The other important aspect as a male health professional in a predominantly female faculty, was the emphasis on treating the whole patient. All our medical lecturers were specialists, and mostly all males. We had excellent grounding in a specific disease or function, such as arthritis, knees, spasms or pneumonia. However, our faculty and profession were strongly female-dominated and still are. All our clinical tutors in the faculty were female and we were taught to always start by assessing and getting to know the patient, a clear lesson in empathy and nurturing. We had to record and write up a white card for every patient. We would always start our goals of treatment with a reminder, 'To gain the confidence and co-operation of the patient.' Treat the patient first, a point I have never forgotten, as in the quote by Sir William Osler at the beginning of this chapter.

This message is now well recognised and is highlighted in Suzanne Chambers' 2021 pivotal book *Facing the Tiger*, dealing with surviving prostate cancer. Emphasis has changed from focussing on the disease (as medicine did in the early days of managing this disease) to acknowledging and addressing the unmet needs, the psycho-social effects on the patient. The patient experience should be the central focus.

Before a man asks the questions that will help him understand and take him to male-hood, he needs to know more about two aspects concerning the basic elements of male-hood. He needs to be aware of how society has formed the idea of manhood and what we expect a man to strive for – the universal qualities of a man. That is, what makes a 'good man'?

This question can be more complex than many assume. One can be a "good man" and quite different in temperament, talents and interests from other men.

While not exhaustive or comprehensive, this list is a compilation of many of the most important widely practiced and culturally expected qualities of manhood according to cultural anthropologists, psychologists and sociologists who have studied the nature of manhood across diverse cultures and time. It is a list of better human qualities which women also fulfil.

- Courage: A man does not shrink from a necessary challenge, regardless of risk. He will face danger, difficulty and self-denial when called upon for the sake of others.
- Step Up: A man is the first one out of his seat (figuratively and literally) when a need arises. He is a problem solver and takes initiative. Passivity is never manly.
- Provide and Protect: A man has learned how and is willing to provide and care for a particular woman (or women) and their common children. He doesn't skip out of his duty. Even if he never marries, he's the kind of person who could do this and provides for others in various ways. As anthropologist David Gilmore concludes, 'A man produces more than he consumes,' and the community benefits from his work and generosity.
- Self-Reliance: A man can stand on his own feet and not need to depend on others for his wellbeing. The Boy Scout motto is 'Be Prepared', because the man doesn't want to have to depend on the preparedness of another. He is not a loner though as he is willing to work with others,
- Honesty and Moral Strength: A man does what is right and calls out others who do not. He deals with others with integrity. Temptation presents itself to every man, but the decisions and actions he takes in light of it significantly determines his manhood. He can be trusted to do what is right when no one is watching. He keeps his word and is dependable to others.

- Tenacity: A man does not easily give up or shrink away in the face of challenge or adversity. He sticks with it and wants to overcome obstacles. 'It can't be done,' doesn't come to him easily.
- Self-Control: A man is aware of the proper limits for himself – his strength, appetites, independence, language and power – and respects them. He calls for others to do the same.
- Under Authority: He is willing to respectfully challenge those in authority when conscience demands, but he is never simply a renegade.
- Shows Respect: A good man shows respect to himself and those he meets, regardless of their station. He looks them in the eye. Gives another man a firm handshake. Offers words of respect such as 'Yes sir/madam,' or 'Thank you, sir.' A man helps others feel valuable.
- Loyalty: A man is loyal to his family, friends and others who are close to him, even at a great price to himself.
- Humility: A man esteems others as valuable and lifts them up. He does not praise himself. He understands the importance of and strength in apologising and asking forgiveness when he has offended or let others down.
- Compassion: This might seem a feminine quality; but is a human quality that has been suppressed in a man, so a man sees the struggles of the weak and those in trouble and readily comes to their aid. This is a moral strength. A man doesn't exploit an innocent person's weakness.
- He lives his character: Lastly, if manhood is a distinct set of character traits, the final quality is that he lives them

out through his actions, and does so conspicuously in the community. To be sure, women may meet all these requirements. However, they tend to do them differently from men and for often different reasons in different situations. This is easily and intuitively recognised by most people. There is no culture in which we would be confused as we observe men and women doing these things for the family.

A man needs to know more about testosterone or androgens. There are many myths and misconceptions that have been sold to us.

Testosterone is a steroid hormone. Androgens is a more scientific name for the family of hormones to which testosterone belongs and is the best known. Hormones are molecules that flow through our circulation and attach to receptors on and in our cells, delivering messages that influence a whole range of body functions. Males and females have testosterone. All foetuses begin life identical in appearance, but at six weeks a testosterone surge in males results in development of the penis. At puberty testosterone production increases further, resulting in the development of male physical (and mental) characteristics.

Testosterone is then responsible for masculine characteristics such as facial and body hair patterns, muscle mass, height, a deep voice. It increases the size of the penis and develops other sexual characteristics. While the majority of testosterone is secreted in the testicles, a small portion (five to ten per cent) is produced by the adrenal glands. When dealing with prostate cancer, testosterone also fuels the growth of certain types of prostate cancer cells, called hormone dependent cells. It also promotes aggressive behaviour, which is probably due to direct stimulation of brain receptors.

There are many myths surrounding testosterone. Even though it is the prototypical masculine hormone, it doesn't mean it is the essence of masculinity. There are many other aspects that make a man. There is also a misconception that our testosterone levels dictate our behaviour.

There is no credible link between high testosterone levels and supposedly masculine traits like risk-taking, assertiveness or bravery. These are mostly learned behaviour or genetic. Nor does it predict your sexual success, unless you have low testosterone (see below) or whether you will be destined to be a domestic violence abuser. It also doesn't predict whether you will live forever or be a good leader. Leaders, like entrepreneurs, are generally born, but they can be taught. Leadership is a set of skills that can be learned by perception, training, practise and experience. A leader is one who comes forward to take a challenge, which has nothing to do with testosterone.

Mistakenly ascribing these changes exclusively to testosterone leads to cultural stereotypes such as men don't cry, men are lecherous, they don't get sick or show pain, men are invincible, they must dominate. It paints testosterone as a mysterious force possessing men, making them do things against their will, including using it as an excuse to prey on women.

To describe somebody as "testosterone-soaked", implying this is a reason for aggressive and violent behaviour, is incorrect. As suggested already, these changes are most likely cultural and developmental which means, fundamentally, we can change the way we think and feel. We just have to find the will – one man at a time.

Testosterone also controls other body functions so a loss in testosterone, either through ageing, disease or treatment for advanced prostate cancer (androgen deprivation therapy) can affect many body systems.

It should also be noted that many studies worldwide indicate men today have less testosterone and sperm in their tanks than our forebears, dropping by about one percentage point a year. The reasons for this are not clear. Reassuringly, most men still have healthy rates of both.

Loss of testosterone ...

- Causes decreased sex drive, or libido, in most men.
- This translates to erectile dysfunction (decreased ability to achieve and maintain an erection) or impotence and loss of desire for sexual activity, especially if castration is performed before puberty, but less so if castration is performed later. Note that eunuchs can gain an erection and enjoy pleasure from sexual stimulation. This caused Chinese emperors to emasculate (cut off their penis) and not just castrate them.
- Influences fertility, the chances to conceive diminish.
- Causes hot flashes, (or flushes) similar to those that women experience during menopause.
- Can cause breast enlargement (also called gynecomastia) and nipple tenderness or sensations.
- Can affect metabolism by slowing it down, causing weight gain around the midsection.
- Can cause cognitive decline and memory loss.
- Can influence mood, leading to reactive depression and lack of sleep.

- Causes a decrease in muscle mass and strength, in turn leading to falls and fractures.
- Causes a decline in bone substance resulting (with a reduction in bone strength), in osteopenia and when more severe, osteoporosis.
- Causes a decrease in energy levels with fatigue being a well-recognised symptom with androgen deprivation therapy.

Any of these signs and symptoms should be a clear and urgent alarm to consult a physician. So, with all this in mind, males have to search for our perception of who we are.

In the next chapter, we will search for the new man – *homo moderna* – modern man or the ideal man. We will call this the avant-garde feather.

CHAPTER TWELVE

The Avant-Garde Feather

'A life without festivity is a long road without an Inn,'
— **Democritus**

Ninety-eight per cent of the 6000 men and women who replied to a questionnaire about what constitutes an ideal man agreed it is an idealist who believes his life is a gift he should revere; that he should leave the world as a better place, and that he should follow the golden rule.

That was twenty years ago when some wondered whether the search for an ideal man, like the quest for the Holy Grail, might be mythic at best and presumptuous at worst; ideal men existed only in platonic heavens or romantic novels. This I contend is incorrect; they exist everywhere. But most of them don't peacock around with bravado.

Perhaps we should leave it there, although that wouldn't do the search justice. Let us probe deeper as things have changed since then.

Looking at the possibilities, if we assess the continuum of a bell curve of types of characters of men, on the left we have the not so good, in the middle seventy per cent we have the average, and on the right, we have the collection of excellent, ideal or exemplary males.

Probably not much good will come of following the ones on the left, the indolent, the wife-beater, the violent and the monstrous man. History is dotted with selfish, narcissistic, ego-driven, power hungry, pathologically toxic masculine men. These are men who advocate wars and odious crime to a level no one else can fathom. Their decisions wreak havoc on humanity and all that comes with it. Each of the following were responsible for murdering millions, Hitler, Stalin, Vlad the Impaler (also known as Vlad Dracula), Pol Pot, Himmler (head of the SS and the brain behind 'the final solution' to the Jewish question), Saddam Hussein, Idi Amin and Genghis Khan.

On the other hand, although women have been shown to have the propensity to be murderous, their crimes are limited to serial killing. The most prolific is said to be the Hungarian Countess Elizabeth Bathory, accused of murdering 650 women (no males) between 1585 and 1610. It may be speculated this limitation could be because psycho-pathologically inclined women, damaged or not, were rarely in a powerful enough position to do worse.

Regardless, criminal anthropologist and author Dr Xanthe Mallet says, 'Women are driven by the same emotions that men are; love, hate, greed. Most crimes come down to one of those. So, you can be the nurturing mother and wife and you can still have those desires and respond to them.'

Such is history's abhorrent record of violence, entrapment and servitude to women; these male characters act as fodder for the whining of the sharp-tongued Katherine of Shakespeare's *Taming of the Shrew*. Kate's response to her mercenary father is a shrewish hatred of men, 'If I be waspish, best beware my sting.'

Her distrust and misandry referred to all men. And I suspect this was because she had a suppressed independent streak and was angry at her non-negotiable situation as a chattel of men. Kate is the "shrew" of the play's title because she does not allow herself to be ordered around by men.

Should we therefore choose our ideal modern man from the great average man, the mediocre man, those who make up the middle seventy per cent of the graph? The ones we don't hear about. These are generally identified as 'good men', the backbone of our society, reliable ones who work for long hours to provide for their family, take the boys to football, the girls to ballet, sit on school P&C committees, then enjoy a few beers with their mates one or two nights a week, a barbie on the weekend, or play golf a couple of times a week. Even though they could be considered as being on autopilot, most would have a sense of purpose, following a familiar pattern, choosing a path to be a good father and husband.

However, their dedicated, stoic attitude in the face of hardship doesn't always prepare them for a life of questioning, of seeking radical change. These are the "reasonable" men, the individuals cited by Irish playwright and political activist George Bernard Shaw when he comments, 'The reasonable man adapts himself to the world; the unreasonable one persists in trying to adapt the world to himself. Therefore, all progress depends on the unreasonable man.'

Which is not completely true. Those men at both extremes of the Gaussian curve (also called "normal" or "bell") could be regarded as unreasonable. Furthermore, governments and institutions now encourage innovation, pushing change. And some attainments by these "unreasonable men" were probably achieved in the spirit of "proving self" or competitiveness.

Most of us are content to live life by these moderate and reasonable maxims, generally productive and secure, and raising confident and resilient children. Until we hit a wall unexpectedly, until we are challenged to think otherwise, then it becomes time to consider whether or not there are alternatives.

The world was recently forced into massive changes to counter the threat from the Covid-19 virus, thereby revealing that large scale culture and behavioural change is possible. Fathers who previously climbed the corporate or commercial ladder, or the majority of men who were content just to do their jobs and marched to the beat of presenteeism, eight-hour days or longer and extreme "busyism", have now been working from home and a great number have stayed home.

As writer Angela Mollard notes, they are now relishing what it is to be involved at a much greater depth in their children's lives. Suddenly the pace of their life has become slower, simpler and more substantial. There is less glamour, glitz and illusion but more earnest conversation over coffee about Pictionary, Scrabble, the creative necessity of gardens, tomatoes and spinach and why the cat, dog and canary don't always get on. There is much less interest in consumerism and materialism and more interest in ecology, recycling, pollution, waste-management and climate change.

These men are also coming to terms with the realisation they don't need to be as focussed on providing as much anymore. Or, as some men do, compete to see who has the biggest mansion, sleekest yacht, fastest car or the need to be an empire builder. 'The man who dies with the most expensive toys wins,' doesn't apply anymore. Or indulge senselessly, as the great hedonist Oscar Wilde says, 'If a thing is worthwhile doing, it's worthwhile overdoing.' Or, to quote Socrates: 'Beware the barrenness of a busy life.'

Along with a growing awareness of unnecessary consumerism and materialism the pressure, to a certain extent, is off. This reprieve will allow the opportunity to explore a more balanced approach to life. Admittedly this may not be the case for those who have lost livelihoods, or those on the breadline already. In some, a simmering anger and rage at their situation still remains.

As writer Mollard has noted, a great deal of these luckier men have regained the neighbourhood and on their morning walks give more than a nod to everyone. They talk now to the natty elderly gentlemen about his roses spilling over the fence, and are mindful of everything and everybody they pass – "mindful" being the operative word. They have lost the intensity for gazing too much inside themselves, forgetting to observe the wider world. From now on, they would be all eyes.

They would have had a chance, and a notion, to comply with another Socrates aphorism, 'The unexamined life is not worth living.'

These men will also wrestle with the idea if it may be time to stop organising society around the warfare system. The other realism concerning modern wars, also stated earlier, is that the individual warrior, as once existed, has little chance to prove his manhood on the battlefield in a one-on-one limited conflict. With total war and the threat of biological warfare or nuclear weapons, man is but another weapon as everyone faces mass destruction.

Pursuing my interests as a military historian, I interviewed hundreds of men and women concerning their war experiences. Their overwhelming and immediate evaluations were generally of the horror and repugnance of war. However, most genuinely valued the camaraderie and bonding which occurs, in what was often part of their formative years. They considered this was one of the most central and pivotal chapters of their life, staying connected to each other for years.

One man commented, 'If you were to sign a paper saying I won't be killed, I would sign up again tomorrow.' Friendships and qualities such as loyalty and discipline stayed with them forever.

But so did heightened experiences of battle and mostly in a negative way, scarring most of them permanently. The anxiety, adrenaline, fear and excitement of one-on-one barbarous conflicts and eventual exhilaration with survival could never be matched or reached in a civil postwar world.

One story stays with me. In 1992, I had been asked to create a sculpture of an Australian Lighthorseman. I was reticent to have him seated on a motionless horse. I wondered whether I could capture him firing while on the back of a galloping horse, a moment of exciting action. I understood this probably wasn't regulatory, so I found WC, a retired Lighthorseman and a country lad from Dubbo, and asked the question.

'Of course,' he said. 'We could all do that, we all did it. We weren't supposed to do it, but we did. Go ahead and do it,' he exhorted with a wicked, defiant glint and smile.

WC had travelled to Egypt in 1915 with the first Australian Infantry Forces. He volunteered to fight as infantry in the horrors of Gallipoli, then took part in "The Great Ride", a three-year desert campaign on horses and camels to push the Turks and Germans out of the Middle East.

In October 1917, he took part in the last cavalry charge in modern warfare. He was one of 800 Lighthorsemen who successfully charged into Turkish embattlements at Beersheba. Strongly entrenched here were 4000 men, sixty machine guns, twenty-four field guns and two German planes which swooped over the battlefield. He described the fear and excitement as he drew his bayonet, the blade flashing in the coppery evening sunlight and thrust it at arm's length while he spurred his horse and galloped at full speed towards them, gambling with life and death. Bullets whizzed past his head, around him he could sense the hysteria and terror mingled with the squeal of stricken horses, the cacophony of troopers yelling wildly – coo-ees and stock yells – and the sound of exploding shells. Shrapnel scattered from air bursts and dust and smoke plumed from ground bursts. To an onlooker, it would have been an incredible spectacle. Thirty-two Australians were killed during the charge.

He remarked it was the most thrilling thing he'd ever done, before or after, and with a laconic smile commented the rest of his life was almost an anticlimax. After the war, he lived a rich, full and productive life. He became a master builder, raised two sons, one an engineer and a Rhodes Scholar, and the other a leading radiologist. By one of life's great coincidences, this son helped me to convene support groups for prostate cancer around Queensland. WC died at ninety-one years.

This experience prompts the suggestion that, for certain personalities, it would not be difficult to imagine how a battlefield high could lead to combat addiction, a well-known phenomenon with defence force personnel.

Contact sport and risk-taking activities have been shown to satisfy a certain amount of this need for the warrior psyche to be quelled. A recent study compared the psychological effects on athletes who engaged in risk-taking activities and contact sports, such as football (all codes), basketball, netball and climbing, with that of non-contact sports such as athletics, swimming, tennis and golf. The contact sport group was shown to be more deeply satisfied and exhilarated at the end of the event.

We recently witnessed the world unite in response to a global pandemic, a common health threat. We may learn from this threat. We may eventually be able to unite swiftly against petty and local aggressors, tyrants and psychopathic despots and act with that same collective will. However, until there is a full de-escalation of war, as alluded to earlier, the sensitive man (or woman) will not be able to stray too far from the dormant warrior under our skin. Society still must support an alert defence system.

Just as importantly, the Covid crisis was a further opportunity to balance the leadership bias. As Elise Stephenson and Susan Harris Rimmer report in *The Interpreter*, gender equality is too often jettisoned when "real problems" arise. They claim that not only is this attitude mistaken, but it can cost lives. They note across their research on gender and Australia's international decision making, one trend really stood out during these times – gender equality is a fair-weather friend quickly abandoned when "real problems" arise, as much as we can have formal policies and rules that institute equality in good times. When a crisis strikes, informal gendered "rules of the game" dominate decision-making and discussion, with women's perspectives and presence often entirely absent.

Further, it is known that women are disproportionally negatively affected by disasters. Crises exploit structural inequalities that affect preparedness, response, impact, number of deaths and recovery. For many Australian women, home is not a place of safety, particularly in times of social distancing and isolation. Domestic violence is already a major health problem, according to the World Health Organisation, with one in three women around the world experiencing physical or sexual violence, let alone other forms of domestic abuse. At least one woman a week is murdered, mostly from an intimate partner, or even a brother or father, protecting the family reputation, or so called "honour".

When women are represented in the highest positions of leadership, they are more likely to look out at the gendered impact of their decisions, even those made in crisis. They can advocate for women and gendered responses, considering children, teachers, childcare workers and aged care workers and school closures. In a crisis, elite men consider counter-terrorism, political violence and the stock market as more important in their areas. Gender equality is not just for good times, a luxury item, but matters in a crisis.

Maybe we will model ourselves on some of the qualities of the high achieving individuals on the right side of the curve. These are often the epitome of the men who change society, the great leaders, the philosophers, entrepreneurs, inventors, scientists, religious men and artists. Men who by their code, commitment and charismatic personality, Mensa intelligence, savant and sometimes sociopathic tendencies pivot the world. Such mythic men with "gentle madness", as exemplified by Cervantes' Don Quixote, when he follows his quest for "the impossible dream".

These are some of my selections for having changed humankind for the better: classical philosophers (Democritus, Socrates), scientists (Galileo, Graham Clarke, inventor of the cochlear implant), political leaders (Churchill, Lincoln, Mandela), religious leaders (Jesus, Gandhi, Buddha), artists (Michelangelo, Da Vinci), explorers (Mawson, Cook), athletes (Jim Thorpe, Michael Phelps), singers (Paul Robeson, Jussi Bjorling), composers (Beethoven, Tchaikovsky, Strauss, Paul McCartney). These are just a few.

Many of these men fit the mould of what would be considered an ideal man, an exemplar. It is worthwhile investigating some of the qualities which set these men aside. We should now examine the benevolent man, the kingly man feather.

CHAPTER THIRTEEN

The Kingly Man Feather

'A good commander is benevolent and unconcerned with fame,'
– Sun Tzu

Throughout history, dreamers have sought them – the ideal men – the exemplars. As Professor John Pearn from the University of Queensland and Associate Professor Richard Franklin, from James Cook University, comment, searching for this degree of idealism, or heroism, can be approached only by an analysis of the altruism (selflessness) and other virtues that underpins it.

Altruism belongs to a distinct, higher ethical category than simply doing your work, your duty. Duty often overlaps with altruism and can compel an individual to reach great heights, but in many instances, it is not regarded as a virtue. Altruism generally involves personal risk. One element of altruism is the presence of that specific quality, undefinable for many, which is variously called "courage", "valour" or "gallantry". Yet it exists at the everyday level – offering a tissue, standing back, bestowing a drink, helping a person with a disability to navigate a staircase.

Lord Moran (1882-1977) wrote in his book, *The Anatomy of Courage* (1945), the essential element of courage is the willpower to handle the instinctive reaction to fear. Courage embodies going beyond self-imposed duty.

It is actually more than overcoming fear. As psychiatrist Jud Brewer explains, to gain courage we have first to deal with the negative effects of anxiety, the close cousin of fear.

Fear is an innate survival mechanism, set up to help us learn what is dangerous and how to avoid it. It is the most primitive survival mechanism we have. Anxiety, on the other hand, is an anti-survival mechanism. Anxiety masks the ability to cope with fear, it masquerades as a promise to help. As American author Arthur Somers Roche put it, 'Anxiety is a thin stream of fear trickling through the mind. If encouraged, it cuts a channel into which all other thoughts are drained.'

Anxiety, ironically, also thwarts learning, making it more difficult to keep facts in your head, confusing your thoughts. An abundance of anxiety drives panic and/or forces our overloaded prefrontal cortex (the thinking and planning part of the brain so important in social behaviour) to shut down.

Once we recognise these negative noisy voices (primitive reactions, anxiety) for what they are, we can then determine if they are really pointing to danger or simply pushing our panic button. Neuroscience has been revelatory about how we behave. Once you deliberately pause a moment and let the amygdala, emotional centre sitting in the temporal lobes of the brain, kick in, you can then think about the situation and name the emotion you are feeling. This allows your cortical brain to activate and make the thinking decisions; only then can you think and you can then turn their volume down. You can then channel this energy into coping with fear.

There is a limit to the usefulness of overcoming fear, to exist in a state of fearlessness. Nicky Barr, an Australian fighter pilot and a double ace during the desert campaign in the Second World War, realised it was probably healthy to possess a certain amount of fear. During my interviews with him he related that at first, he was often mesmerised by people who showed no fear. He appreciated this "fearless" style did wondrous things for morale and in a way encouraged leadership qualities in others.

However, he learned to be critical of such individuals as he could see they possessed a tendency towards a reckless attitude towards life, with the potential to unnecessarily endanger themselves as well as the rest of the squadron. In effect, he considered they lacked a sensitivity that was necessary for war and survival. He considered this fearlessness could be dangerous when allowed to dominate. Split-second reactions, so important in combat, were aided by this sensitivity born of fear.

The situation is little different when one has to make a decision to step up and be counted, particularly in acts of altruism.

The baseline or strategic background in which altruistic acts are performed is the broad generic acceptance of the ethic of the biblical story of the Good Samaritan, or the underlying secular humanistic ethic of the Golden Rule, treating others as you would wish to be treated yourself. It is considered these altruistic acts are performed by individuals with a prior higher ethics, learned primarily in childhood, but reinforced in adult life. Altruism also enlists other virtues as endurance, loyalty and honesty.

In everyday life, we imagine that we would, or should, do everything we can do to help someone in trouble. Most individuals with an upbringing in the Judeo-Christian, Buddhist, Hindu, Muslim or secular Humanist tradition would imagine, in a non-specific way, that they would step forward and do the right thing if they could help.

Ernest Becker (1924-1974), a cultural anthropologist and professor at Berkeley University in California, sought such idealism. In his 1973 book, *The Denial of Death*, published a year before his own death, and for which he was awarded the Pulitzer Prize two months after his death by cancer at forty-nine, discusses this theme.

As he drew on the inevitability of his own death, he spoke of the intellectual and moral courage needed by good men to think clearly about the nature of injustice. And the need to confront the terrifying awareness of the primitive, animalistic character seething under our skin. Be it criminal behaviour, law, health, scientific acknowledgement or personal freedoms – racial, gender or religious – the hero's path in the world is bound to be filled with conflict. He will be the one who will stand and be counted, displaying feelings of moral indignation. He will try to create change because he can. And I quote Becker, 'The most exalted type of heroism involves feelings that one has lived to some purpose that transcends one.'

Becker emboldens us to feel heroic in ways that can help to bring about a better world.

We should search further. What exactly do we mean by the expression "heroic" or indeed, "the heroic ideal?" I suppose we mean the picture of what a perfect hero should be like, and this raises the question of what we mean by "hero", and is this and the "ideal" concept qualities that are unchanging through time?'

Let us travel back as far as Homer's *The Iliad*, the story of the siege of Troy, sparkling with the mythical heroes Achilles, Ulysses and Hector, then to the Hellenic period of Alexander the Great

(356-323 BC), the ultimate Greek hero who amassed the most extensive empire that the world had seen. It was useful to listen to Emeritus Professor Bob Milns, former head of the classics department at the University of Queensland.

Reinforcing what we have already considered about males and fighting, Milns suggests one quality of the hero that has survived across the ages is that of outstanding excellence in warfare. This may be as an individual fighter or as a successful and bold leader of fighters, especially where the conquest of others and acquisition of territory is concerned (and the successful repelling of would-be conquerors).

I have found this concept was still strong until recent times. As military writer Walter J Boyne has noted in his book *Aces in Command* (2001), over the years three enduring warrior symbols capture the public's imagination – the cocky, aggressive fighter pilot ace, the knight in shining armour and the laconic, gun-toting cowboy. Yet, I believe this is not necessarily so for the current generation. Modern heroes such as Barack Obama, Chuck Feeney, Bill Gates, Dick Smith and Neil Armstrong present different role models.

Alexander the Great had a vision, a dream of uniting a new realm, rooted in conquest, but flourishing with peace and enlightenment to join nations together. Ideas as well as merchandise would be exchanged. He welded the majority of three continents into a single entity, while allowing their constituents to maintain their religious and cultural institutions.

He did this by turns charismatic and ruthless, brilliant and power hungry, diplomatic and bloodthirsty. To achieve his aims, thousands of soldiers and civilians died or were enslaved, women raped and cities pillaged and razed.

It is difficult to balance such ambition from ego-driven psychopathic and narcissist conquerors with the potential positive effects of unification. And there are other qualities which tend to be associated with heroic stature that Alexander did not heed.

One quality he did not possess was the ability to accept pertinent pieces of advice from his teachers. Alexander's teacher was Aristotle, one of the greatest of the early philosophers. Aristotle's mentor, in turn, was Plato, a philosopher who had recorded his teacher Socrates' teachings, among them what was known as *The Socratic Dialogues*. Socrates detested war and challenged leaders to discuss every situation and conflict ad-infinitum, if necessary, before warfare.

Milns suggests these Socratic features may be summed up in the Greek word "megalopsychia", which means "greatness of soul" and implies such qualities as generosity to friends and defeated enemies; mercy towards the weaker; absolute loyalty to one's comrades; frank and open behaviour, which never hides behind subterfuge; and perhaps above all a burning desire to achieve immortality through one's glorious deeds. Many of these qualities are those of what is often referred to as The Kingly Man, one who is kingly because he displays greatness of soul and heroic qualities.

Alexander and most conquerors do not meet these requirements. Milns is strong in his condemnation. There is little to display in the career of Alexander that can be shown to have been intended for the well-being of his subjects. There was much to show he was deeply concerned with himself and promoting his own glory. For too long the world has allowed itself to be mesmerised and dazzled by the aggressive and murderous activities of a handful of self-centred glory-seekers and has measured achievements by the number of innocent people slaughtered and the amount of alien territory violently seized.

The old male bonding activities of war, sport, drinking, hunting, shooting, fishing and female conquests are no longer appropriate for what should define a modern male. True virility is embedded in virtues like loyalty, courage and altruism.

So, my troupe of ideal men, exemplars, or heroes, will be self-actualised fierce men, daring, with courage and cunning, men who will rise in considered judgement. Instead of entering the arena with swords and guns, they will wrestle with their intellect, their tongues and their keyboards. They will joust with the mystery of injustice in its many guises. They will become warriors in defence of inequalities which impact on our quality of life. They will become protectors of the powerless and healers of the overwhelmed, fulfilling a role once used to protect the tribe.

These principles were also enshrined by religious leaders who led by example, costing both Jesus and Gandhi their lives. Regardless whether you consider yourself to be a true believer in the life, death and resurrection of the son of God, or you have a scholar's quest for the historical non-supernatural Jesus, it was his defining message that was important. His unwavering direction and final actions for us to accept unconditional love, reverberate and inspire through the centuries. However, the patriarchal church founded in his name, the largest corporate institution in history, does not always reflect his simple words and has some distance to go before it is seen as a true leader of gender equality.

I've always liked Martin Luther King Jr's statement, 'The ultimate measure of a man is not where he stands in moments of comfort and convenience, but where he stands at times of challenge and controversy.'

Regarding the military, there were probably as many reasons for joining the military as there were men or women but eventually, like so many service personnel in any war, certain individuals are called upon to do the killing or be killed themselves – the bottom line for any war.

Courage emerges at these times in all its forms and gradations. To have the fortitude, the will and the spirit to persevere, to fight on when the outlook is seemingly desperate, when the perceived odds of surviving are slim, surely requires a special quality.

These qualities are often used to describe the Australian soldier. They are summed up by the inscription of the four monumental pillars erected on the site of the 1942 pivotal battle at Isurava on the Kokoda Track in New Guinea – Courage, Endurance, Mateship and Sacrifice.

You probably get my drift. These outstanding qualities of the kingly man, the exemplar male, are also reflected in the arts, explorers, athletes, dancers, celebrities, singers and composers, in fact every endeavour in which human beings take part. Heroic men stand up and are counted in any sphere.

In the early chapters of this book, I endeavoured to construct an historic blueprint of from where males evolved and where, as a broad gender, we sit now.

Let us travel on a journey and look at a roadmap to build our modern man, our new man, our "Ideal Man".

CHAPTER FOURTEEN

The Odyssean Feather – Roadmap for an Odyssey

'A man must go on a quest
To discover the sacred fire
In the sanctuary of his own belly
To ignite the flame in his heart
To fuel the blaze in the hearth
To rekindle his ardour for the earth,'
– **Sam Keen**

When I was at my lowest ebb and began this journey, I needed to prepare a roadmap to help with the milestones and directions. I realised I had hit the wall, so to address this epiphany, I pushed the starter button and began my odyssey.

As the frontiers opened up, I found this adventure had the markings of the universal story, the common theme of the bestselling stories of all time, from Troy to Star Wars, the archetypical "myth of the hero". A boy grows up in a village, content and unquestioning with the life and traditions he has inherited. He is then threatened by an outside force. This could be marauding conquerors, criminals or bacteria. Or it could be an internal force, even his own demons.

Chapter Fourteen The Odyssean Feather – Roadmap for an Odyssey

The boy leaves the comfort of the village, or the whirrings and prison of his mind, to confront the menace. In the process he experiences a legion of adventures, some painful, some leading to loss. Eventually he conquers great adversaries and returns to the village a man. His view of life is considerably transformed and he is imbued with a degree of insight and wisdom. He achieves an apotheosis.

The first challenge on my journey was to search for the possibility and extent of my own denial. This was in regard to my own invincibility and my perceived position of dominance.

As part of this process, some men may be disinterested in, or resistant to, efforts to involve themselves in progressive change. This is probably because some of us may have widespread negative attitudes which are hard-wired and ingrained.

So, it is granted a certain number of men may not be able to, or willing, to change. These men will predominately be contained in the special bracket of 'entitled', those who display a glaring hypocrisy or a casual double standard. Those who treat misogyny not so much as virulent woman-hating, but as a more systemic social enforcement mechanism, a way to keep women in their place in their patriarchal world.

As the philosopher Kate Manne writes in her book *Entitled*, 'An illegitimate sense of male entitlement gives rise to a wide range of misogynistic behaviour. When a woman fails to give a man what he's supposedly owed – admiration, sex and consent; a home where someone else uncomplainingly does most of the child care and housekeeping – she will often face punishment and reprisal.' Some of these things are 'feminine-coded', she writes. Others, like power and knowledge, are typically reserved as a masculine prerogative.

This charter is particularly striking when a man, for whatever reason, contemplates having an affair. He may rationalise his deception in many ways, convincing himself that if he was honest with his partner it could disrupt other family members or destabilise his work or the couple's social status. Keep it quiet – okay to cheat.

It therefore becomes onerous to judge particular potential ideal men in the community when eminent figureheads and inspirational role models display their lack of integrity at a personal level. Their credibility should be challenged. Such men as Luciano Pavarotti, one of the most talented singers in history, often used his charm and philanthropy as a Trojan horse to legitimise his well-known philandering. Presidents of the USA, such as Bill Clinton, who had an affair with an intern (and with many others), "because he could", and John F Kennedy, who fabricated a fairy-tale image of himself while reigning over the new Camelot, was a serial womaniser. His charisma convinced the entire White House staff to be complicit, for them all to impute dishonesty. Yet how do you balance these luminaries' often great legacies against their infidelities?

At the start of our journey, it is important we internalise and overcome this. The implication here is that significant community change may not happen in our lifetime, we may have to work for generational change. We will have to educate not just ourselves, but also the next generation.

As James Prochaske from the University of Rhode Island has noted, it can be a difficult process to change behaviour, any behaviour. He suggests that individually making a behaviour change should be approached as if you were getting ready for a major surgery. It requires a great amount of preplanning; you need to develop an action plan. It requires support from family and friends and you should consider this plan your number one priority.

As it requires great mental attention choose a time when there is nothing else within your control to take precedence. Preferably not a time when you are making marital change, job change, major vacation, getting ready to move house etc. Healthy behaviour change is that difficult and it is that important.

As part of your strategy, you may need to change your environment, where you live and with whom you work. This will include your friends.

Finally, give yourself every opportunity to create a successful odyssey, journey by assessing the friends around you. Choose your friends, your tribe, carefully. Remove yourself from clinging ones who drain you, who "dump" on you and have a generally negative, depressive, pessimistic and sceptical view of life. This is not easy, but if you surround yourself with brilliant, ambitious, positive, optimistic and inspiring people, your behaviour will begin to change. You will find a new zest for life.

CHAPTER FIFTEEN

The Futuristic Feather

'The reality we live in is the construct of our ancestors; the reality our children will live in, will be the construct of our actions.'
— Abhyit Naskar

I don't intend to look too seriously at some of the long-term projections concerning the future of males, such as the damning evidence which suggests we are slowly losing our Y chromosome. The Y chromosome is the "male determining gene", the one which causes testes to form in the embryo, to allow us to become male. Jenny Graves, a distinguished professor of genetics at La Trobe University, Melbourne, has found verification that the human Y chromosome is degenerating and may disappear in a few million years, leading to our own species extinction unless we evolve a new sex gene. She reports the good news that two branches of rodents have already lost their Y chromosome and have adapted and lived to tell the tale.

Graves adds that evolution of a new sex determining gene comes with risks. What if more than a new system evolves in different parts of the world? A war of the sex genes could lead to the separation of new species, so if aliens visited Earth in eleven million years they might find no humans, or several different human species, kept apart by their different sex determination systems.

Even more urgent, Bryan Sykes, an Oxford University professor in genetics, has cut the extinction time considerably. He has hypothesised that within 5000 generations, 125,000 years, reproduction associated with the Y chromosome will become extinct.

Either way I don't think we should be concerning ourselves too much with these revelations just yet. What is obvious is that at this stage there has been a transitioning of perspective from one where males have traditionally perceived themselves to be the protectors, the providers and procreators, to one where we are now confronting a startling different reality.

Our simplistic historical role of existing within the boundaries of these three Ps has been seriously eroded, perhaps forever.

For most of us, coming to terms with this variation has not been easy. I suspect the shift became obvious initially at the end of the nineteenth century with female enlightenment, education and the suffragette movement, forcing men to look at themselves and particularly their stance on equality – to "unshackle the chains of yesteryear". The next large change possibly came from the introduction of the oral contraceptive pill in the 1950s. This dramatically transformed generations, giving women incredible freedom and reproductive autonomy. And in recent times, the #MeToo movement and its offshoots have made an indelible impression on male-female relationships.

How should modern males embrace this situation? There are many suggestions which I will touch on in the following chapters but first we have to begin by seeing everything through the lens of accepting gender equality.

Let me give you an example from my own experience as to

how society, including myself, was ideologically indoctrinated into concluding that males should be dominant.

I started my first full-time job in 1961, fifteen years after the end of the Second World War had finished. Even though the feminist movement had well-started, gender inequality and subsequent injustices were still strongly in place.

I began work as a clerk in a Public Service Department where most of the clerks were men, either with a senior pass (Grade 12) or similar standard. There was a large typist pool with about 400 young women aged from sixteen to about twenty-five, all with a junior standard education (Grade 10). In that era, it was still considered very unimportant for women to have a higher education. Most of them did a home economics course to prepare them for domesticity. What I noticed and accepted as normal was that the women received substantially less pay than the males, even if doing the same job. What was even more bizarre, and in retrospect grossly unfair, was that the women had to leave work once they were married and were not eligible for superannuation.

In November 1965 this changed when Prime Minister Harold Holt decreed it would now be legal for married women to work in the public service. As ABC writer Annabel Crabb scathingly comments, 'The principle behind the law was twofold. First, before then, it was felt that a female public servant who got married would no longer be capable of doing her job, given the notorious female incapacity to perform any other sensible function simultaneously with the task of gestation, curtain selection or the cooking of a chop.

'There was, moreover, an ancillary disinclination to allow women who had snared a lifelong financial benefactor (a husband) to double-dip by holding down a paid job that should by rights go either to a man or to a spinster who needed occupation to stave off the pangs of despair, plus enough money for cat food.'

There was also a strong drinking culture among the staff in those days. After work, the men would network at the local pub, building on relationships and cementing career pathways. Women were not allowed into bars, only into the ladies' lounge, generally a room next door with comfortable chairs, further disadvantaging them. They were finally allowed into bars in Australia in the 1970s, 1969 in Queensland.

Some years later, I attended the University of Queensland and graduated as a physiotherapist in 1966. There I met my wife, a speech therapist, one of the first in the state. Her father was an enlightened El Alamein veteran and her parents were determined their four daughters and son would have access to the highest education. After our honeymoon and coming home after our respective first day at work, we struck a problem. As a priority, my wife had been a keen student and had never really been taught how to cook. And, of course, nor could I. She straight away offered to attend cooking courses. It never occurred to me that I should do that. And I look back in amazement now that I accepted her doing the ironing (including mine) washing and house cleaning.

Such was the strength of the embedded stereotype roles of the day. I must add though, I fell into my stereotypical role of looking after the yard, car, rubbish, cutting the wood and later maintaining the pool, without a whimper. That's what males did. It never occurred to me my wife may have preferred to do those assignments. (She wouldn't have, I know now).

It wasn't until twenty-five-years later, after our children left home and my wife founded a charity to teach children who are deaf to listen and to speak that these roles changed. When my wife began PhD studies, for viability and out of necessity I was given an opportunity to learn to cook. I am now an adequate preparer of food and regret the years of creative culinary experiences I missed out on, and we now share the ironing and cleaning.

My son and daughter's generation has broken down the barriers a great deal more. My son is an excellent cook and helps care and educate his son while working at home in IT with his partner, a barrister. My daughter has two degrees and had a full-time creative career in music before her marriage, and now is a full-time housemother for her three children. My grandchildrens' generation has changed the definition of gender roles again, as we have already discerned.

So the following sentence is the basis for the rest of the book – it is where the futuristic feather should spring from;

Real change means accepting that a female is a human being who should enjoy exactly the same rights as a male.

Period!

Gender equality means women and men enjoy the same status. To think otherwise is simply bigotry. Society demands a different type of male and a different type of leader, one who is inclusive, collegial, collaborative and encourages creativity, benevolence, innovation and independence.

I have stressed this concept earlier – men, masculinity and even fatherhood have changed in recent times. Fathers can be straight or gay, married or single, adoptive or step, stay-at-home or working. It is therefore important to promote gender equality. A suggestion – try to support a gender equality education and promotion campaign with the emphasis on engaging men and boys because the best place to start is with educating young men.

Gender equity, on the other hand, recognises that to be fair different steps may be needed to create fair and equal outcomes. This is because of the differences in women's and men's lives as well as historical disadvantages. In the business world particularly, the Merle Pledge, is a very worthwhile activity with which to be acquainted and to act out.

Merle Thornton is an Australian feminist activist and author. She is best known for her 1965 action at the Regatta Hotel in Toowong, Brisbane, where she and Rosalie Bogner famously chained themselves to a bar rail to protest at the exclusion of serving women in public bars in Queensland. She helped establish the first women's studies course at the University of Queensland in 1973 and developed what is known as the Merle Pledge.

Many high-profile conferences, events, task forces and media outlets lack gender balance, despite there often being no shortage of qualified women to contribute.

The Merle Pledge was created for university staff to address and uphold the lack of gender balance at conferences and events, requesting gender equity as a condition of their participation on panels and at conferences. In 2020 the University of Queensland adapted and initiated the pledge concept for panel use.

In essence, the pledge calls for the individual to commit to,

- Increasing the visibility and contribution of women in public and professional forums.
- Advocating the gender balance and diversity in all professional events, panels and conferences.
- Actively encouraging and supporting the voices of women

and when attending or organising panel sessions and conferences make it known to colleagues that you stand for gender equality and you will only support, attend and organise events organised where a gender diverse panel or line-up of speakers is offered (or all reasonable attempts have been made).

- Question the composition of panellists and speakers and reserve their right to withdraw from events, even at the last minute, if gender balance and diversity are not achieved.

For further information about the Merle Pledge, visit https://sciencegenderequity.org.au

CHAPTER SIXTEEN

The Beseeching Feather – Ask for Help

'Life isn't about waiting for the storm to pass... it's learning to dance in the rain,'
– **Vivian Green**

Another direct difficulty which has risen from males presuming they need to be seen as being in charge has been resistance to asking for help or advice concerning almost anything. It has been important for us to be appreciated as independent and infallible leaders.

Asking for help is a sign of strength. The beseeching feather, asking for help, is one of the most important feathers we can add to our display. In a recent feature article in the *Sport Health Journal* (Vol 38, issue 2, 2021) concerning cultural influences and barriers to elite athletes seeking treatment for mental health disorders, it was reported elite athletes often believe mental health symptoms and disorders are a sign of weakness, or report stigma associated with them. Several factors are associated with negative attitudes about seeking help for mental health treatment. These include identification as male, hypermasculinity, younger age, Black (versus Caucasian) race, United States (versus European) nationality, gender role conflicts and participation in physical contact sports.

Men will get sick like everyone else; disease does not favour gender. This is particularly important for the macho (and stoic) male to understand. It is not all right to play sport with broken bones, to deny you are in pain, to swagger in defiance of authority and common sense. It is also not all right to blindly fight to remain at the top of the pecking order by aggression, extreme toughness, bullying and displaying autocratic tendencies. It is also not all right to create or to follow aggressive tribal rituals, demanding blind allegiance.

It is easy to act tough by pretending that problems don't exist. It takes courage and strength to admit you might need help, regardless of whether you have mental health problems or a painful knee.

The same can be said when males are in leadership roles. Society now demands leaders who are collaborative and can share with decision making. Most effective leaders these days are facilitators, not autocratic controllers.

With reference to mental health, it is not a sign of weakness to have down times – to be depressed.

It is extremely important to recognise that men and their partners understand the consequences of not identifying and addressing depression. There is a quiet crisis in Australia right now. The latest figures (from Griffith University in Queensland's 2020 annual report) reveal more than five men aged thirty-five to thirty-nine are killing themselves every week in Queensland alone, in a male midlife suicide dilemma.

To a partner, the warning signs are not always obvious, particularly with a middle-aged man. At this stage of his life, as mentioned earlier, he may be stoically dealing with financial issues, work pressure and stress, an expanding family, lack of time for exercise and other health issues, tired and dealing with the external perception of the world that he may not be coping. There are other reasons, also not so obvious – shame, relationships, addiction, careers and self-worth.

While in this darkest corner of their life, they may feel they are an unfixable burden on themselves and others. This may particularly be the case with older men where body systems are breaking down and pain and loss of independence is an everyday tribulation.

As already mentioned in the introduction, men aged eighty-five and older have the highest suicide rates in Australia, more than three times the average (Australian Bureau of Statistics).

The signs to look for are being moody, irrational, confused, unable to switch off and concerned about the future. He may also become withdrawn, changing his online behaviour, losing interest in what he used to love, unable to concentrate and become less interested in his personal appearance and hygiene. His sleep patterns may also change, and he may behave recklessly.

This is the stage where depression can affect the chemicals of your brain and it is not always a situation that an individual may have control over. The brain gets taken to such a dark place that it is difficult to ask for help.

A lot of men still don't want to talk about mental health issues – there is a sustained culture of silence and stigma here.

Suicide ideation becomes a real option, which brings up another aspect. A relative or friend may angrily consider that the man's suicidal actions have been selfish and judge him harshly. Stop for a moment and consider that it may be quite unfair for a rational mind to adjudicate on the functioning of a dysfunctional, irrational mind.

Asking, 'Are you okay?' is always an excellent starting point and is often an important circuit-breaker. Mention specific things in their behaviour which prompted you to ask, 'You seemed more quiet than usual of late,' or such like. But it should be taken further.

There is often resistance by friends to do this, as friends may be concerned that they aren't qualified like a doctor. However, every human being is qualified to ask someone if they are okay. The friend can fear, wrongly, that if they mention the word suicide it is going to put the idea into their heads, which is not the case at all.

As John Brogden, patron of Lifeline Australia, comments, all their experience and research shows that asking direct questions such as: 'Are you feeling suicidal, do you want to kill yourself, do you want to hurt yourself?' is the best way to cut through. A direct question. If they say 'Yes,' and open up, then encourage action. Tap into your wider network of friends, family and medical professionals. Get help by calling a doctor, call Lifeline or accompany them to an emergency department. Do not leave them. Treat them the same way you would treat someone who had a heart attack in front of you.

Make sure you follow up. According to findings by Movember (a global movement to raise awareness for men's health) forty-five per cent of men drop out early after seeking professional help.

From my perspective, in the early days of my cancer diagnosis, when I was aberrantly spiralling into reactive depressive cycles I often dallied with thoughts of suicide. In those dark days, my wife was my rock. However, I would have welcomed a medical professional reaching out and asking if I was okay and acknowledging the medical issues.

It wasn't until I started my own prostate cancer support group and invited specialist speakers that I became aware of, and was able to address, these psycho-social and other unmet needs.

Another situation which seems to hit men hard can be retiring from an elite sport or being discharged from the miliary. While some can thrive and never look back by finding a new career and lifestyle, others can spiral downward with mental health issues and even suicide. They can find themselves on an emotional roller coaster before eventually finding their feet as ordinary civilians.

There can be a tremendous loss of identity, as well as sense of purpose, motivation and resilience. As Dan Pronk notes in his book, *The Resilience Shield*, you can also lose your tribe. The military is the ultimate tribe, bringing members together in tight-knit groups that share bonding experiences, including training, combat and loss of team mates. To lose this support, from the ones who understand you the most, can be devastating.

No less, the same for elite sportspersons. They can also spend years together, training for a common goal, often dealing with injuries and pressure from coaches, clubs, media, sponsors and the public. This is regardless of whether you are a member of a national sporting team, rugby for instance, or you are training for an individual event as part of an athletics or swimming squad.

Suddenly, for athletes and miliary personnel alike, civilian life can be boring. After working and training, competing under extreme levels of occupational stress with high functioning motivated people, adjustment to a quieter society may take some recalibration. It is pivotal that there is an opportunity to consult specialists and psychologists towards changing these concepts. Ideally, this should be done very early in their sporting (or military) careers, particularly as some elite athletes can do, before they have the potential to develop an exaggerated view of themselves.

Keeping in touch with sport or military mates can be useful. Changing values must also be taught. It takes years to be a top athlete, or military person, so it may take time to regulate – give yourself some years to adjust. But, as this chapter is titled, if you are struggling – 'Ask for help.'

Another valid way to ask for help is to find support from family, friends or other individuals or groups going through similar circumstances. The next chapter aims to help you take advantage of this concept.

CHAPTER SEVENTEEN

The feather of the stout-hearted men – find a support group

'We are all healers of each other,'
– Rachel Naomi Remen MD

A consistent pattern of evidence over a long period of time confirms the effectiveness of support groups for people coping with specific challenges. Whether dealing with a chronic illness, emotional problem, loneliness, life transition or wanting to enhance your health and wellbeing, joining a community group of people in the same situation can help fill the void.

A men's support group or men's health support group are forums where men can share personal stories, express emotions and be heard in an atmosphere of non-judgmental acceptance, understanding and encouragement. A sense of loss and/or isolation can be created when men have a sudden change in life direction. This could be retirement, career ceiling reached, retrenchment, disability, sickness, divorce, a marriage under stress or broken down or death of a partner.. These can also trigger a need to seek assistance.

Zac Seidler, a clinical psychologist and director of mental health training at Movember, the annual November fundraiser for men's health issues, says, 'If you can help men proactively – and not reactively – understand and respond to their emotional lives before a crisis arises, we'll have well-adjusted respectful men.' (quoted by Greg Callaghan, *The Australian*, 6 May 2023).

Such groups as Men's Sheds Australia were created for this reason. The sheds offer an opportunity for disconnected older men to reconnect with their peers. One of the first groups in Australia was started in Broken Hill in the 1980s. Another started in Sydney's Lane Cove in 1988 as a community men's shed. Other groups started spontaneously around Australia so that by 2005, there were an estimated 200 Men's Sheds operating in Australia. By 2021 there were almost a thousand, totalling thousands of active members.

Its social connection and a sense of purpose which drives men to meet where they can put on a kettle and have a chat, or get to work on a project where they will work shoulder to shoulder. The sheds provide a male-only space for craftwork (carpentry etc), social interaction, hobbies, playing video-games, congregating with friends or just having coffee with a mate. The concept reflects best-practice in men's health promotion.

But this isn't your regular mateship. This is the kind that helps improve social wellbeing and saves the lives of those who have suffered deeply from loneliness and heartache. They are now researching the link between isolation, frailty and mental health.

There are now many other men's groups throughout Australia, often under the banner of Men's Health. Such entities as Men's Wellbeing, Pit Stop, Men's Work projects, Men's Health and Wellbeing, Men Care Too (an organisation that supports male carers), Centre for Men and Sydney Men's Festival. These groups regularly come together nationally in the Gatherings of Men's

Gathering, where events and activities for men are discussed. This includes Men's Health Week, held every June. Men's Health Week started in the USA in 1994 to heighten awareness of preventable health problems such as cardiac, diabetes, cancers and mental health, including suicide. One of three men experience some kind of reproductive or sexual health problem.

For further information and access to many varied men's groups contact Australian Men's Health Forum, the peak body for men's health in Australia at https:/www.amhf.org.au

Or email admin@amhf.org.au

In this context, the organisation Healthy Male – Andrology Australia is a valid, scientifically-based source of information on men's health and is highly recommended. Contact: Healthymale.org.au.

There are also specific support groups for particular health problems. As mentioned, in 1996, I started one of the first support groups for prostate cancer in Australia. At that stage, I could find no research on prostate cancer in Australia, and no other men to talk to, and no real help to deal with the side-effects of treatment.

With other fledgling groups around Australia, in that same year we formed the Prostate Cancer Foundation of Australia (PCFA), the peak consumer body for prostate cancer in Australia. Our Brisbane group grew to be one of the largest in Australia, hosting 1000 members and there are now 170 such groups nationally.

I morphed into the role as convenor. From the beginning, I approached the best health professionals who could deliver up-to-date evidenced-based information on all aspects of prostate cancer, revisiting and upgrading these and other topics as they became relevant on an annual basis. Over the years, I have organised some 230 meetings at which this information was delivered and eventually shared with all Queensland support groups and the national body PCFA. This was the first time any men's health groups had really existed in Australia and the men (and their partners) realised this was a safe and enclosed environment to discuss their health and their vulnerabilities.

In this non-judgmental forum, men could lower their defences. They could demonstrate their anger, shame and feelings of loss, grief and guilt associated with their diagnosis, their struggle with relationships, their difficulties dealing with erectile dysfunction, incontinence and the many other side-effects of treatment, particularly the losses from treatment of advanced prostate cancer. Some cried, sobbed and readily asked for and accepted assistance.

As friendships and trust grew, an interesting phenomenon occurred. These men felt confident to discuss other frailties, to reveal their loneliness, frustrations, degenerative conditions, co-morbidities with ageing and simply share what it means to be a man to the only people who really understand their situation from a similar perspective – other men. This does not dismiss the ability and willingness of women to appreciate the difficulties encountered by men. In the process, they have not only taken control of their own lives and health care, along with other support groups, they have driven the development of the men's health movement in Australia.

There are often musically inclined people in our group and we occasionally have sing-alongs, which are fun and promote bonding. We chose as our theme song *Stout Hearted Men* by Sigmund Romberg and Oscar Hammerstein II for the 1927 operetta *The New Moon*..

Chapter Seventeen   The feather of the stout-hearted men – find a support group

> Give me some men
> Who are stout-hearted men,
> Who will fight for the right they adore.
> Start me with ten
> Who are stout-hearted men,
> And I'll soon give you
> Ten thousand more.
> Shoulder to shoulder,
> And bolder and bolder,
> They grow as they go to the fore,
> Then there's nothing in the world
> Can halt or mar a plan,
> When stout-hearted men
> Can stick together man to man.

The song was pertinent to us as we started our group with about ten men and grew to 10,000 around Australia as PCFA (Prostate Cancer Foundation of Australia).

As information and support for men with prostate cancer became more readily available these support groups often evolved, particularly in rural areas, into important social groups for men and their extended families.

Just as importantly, as internationally esteemed researcher and president of the Union for International Cancer Control (UICC) and former CEO and chef de mission and head of research of PCFA, Professor Jeff Dunn comments, 'Over the past thirty years, prostate cancer survival rates have increased from fifty-eight to ninety-five per cent, which is a remarkable achievement in the Australian context. This is a credit to rapid advancements in research, awareness and support for patients.'

Eventually, two survivors of prostate cancer, politicians Jim Lloyd, from New South Wales (the national support groups' executive for PCFA) and Wayne Swan from Queensland (who launched my book on prostate cancer, *Conquering Incontinence* in 2003), placed a private members' Bill to Parliament. This led in May 2010 to the government releasing the first national male health policy and providing $16.7 million to fund the policy. This instantly changed the validity of acceptance of support for men. Funding immediately assisted a great number of organisations including Men's Sheds and men struggling with prostate cancer.

No man shall ever be alone again. Let him wear this feather with sartorial elegance and pride.

CHAPTER EIGHTEEN

The Loving Feather – Relationships

'A successful relationship requires falling in love many times; always with the same person,'
– **Mignon McLaughlin**

Why do men place such emphasis on sex? From some women's point of view, it would appear we place too much emphasis on it.

When considering relationships, I believe that there is a fault with male society's fixation with penetrative sex. This is particularly true for the macho male. I don't believe we will find the proof of our masculinity here. These actions restrict the whole range of activity which humans crave, such as intimacy and sensual contact. Sex may bring instant pleasure or joy, but not identity of manhood.

Because we have learned to measure our manhood by things that can be quantified, how much money, how big is your empire, your house, how sporty and powerful is your car, how many lovers you have, or how much weight you can lift, we have become poor in experiencing the richness of the small daily pleasures that must be savoured moment by moment.

Why do men place such emphasis on penetration and a quick

exciting climax as being the major event in the sex encounter? You have only to look back to the singular model he knows, the only one that males have known for thousands of years. It is the period when men's primeval need and their egos became nearly inseparable from their penises. Male identity revolves around the penis in a way that female identity does not revolve around the vagina.

A popular book on the subject – *The Ugly Truth about Men*, by Tom Carey, 1992 – has stated that, like it or not, one of the ugly truths about men is that they are thinking about some aspect of sex much of the time, as often as every four minutes, whereas women apparently only think about sex four times a day or less.

Once again, we shouldn't be too surprised if we look at our primal ancestry. As mentioned earlier, Zarin Machanda, a primatologist at Tufts University who has spent nearly twenty years studying the wild chimps of Uganda's Kibale National Park, states that male chimp's sexual appetite is rapacious. As reported in the April 2021 edition of *Men's Health*, Machanda comments, 'They want sex constantly and get it constantly, up to twelve times a day, each encounter lasting a frantic seven to ten seconds. The females, generally speaking, dare not deny them.'

On the other hand, bonobos, a close relative of the chimp who shared the same ancestor until a million years ago, are far more tolerant, more social and peace keeping. They are, however, inordinately sexual. Instead of releasing tension by fighting, they couple repeatedly. They have been labelled as the most sex-crazed mammals of all time. As well as pleasure, sex is a social tool. It reaffirms common bonds, relieves tension and keeps the peace. Importantly, alpha females run the bonobo tribe, whereas males rule the chimp tribes.

Added to this revelation, with the advent of easily accessible online pornography, particularly for males, if there are no checks and balances on these thoughts and images it is not difficult to understand how it may lead to unrealistic expectations and sexualised behaviour. For any age group, porn is easily accessed before breakfast, lunch time, after school or work or on the bus. This unrelenting stimulation can develop into an excessive preoccupation with sexual fantasies and urges, leading to objectification and probable addiction, treating the woman as an object, valuing the woman exclusively on the basis of her body, rather than on her full identity.

How did this difference start? Probably back to the boy and his first sexual initiation, the one he unexpectedly discovered in his sleep – wet dreams. Up until this stage, a boy's life revolved around what the ancient fourth century philosopher Kalidasi promised in his *Salutation to the Dawn*:

> Salutation to the Dawn.
> Look to this day,
> For it is life, the very life of life,
> In its brief course lie all the
> Varieties and realities of your existence,
> The bliss of growth,
> The glory of action,
> The splendour of beauty;
> For yesterday is but a dream,
> And tomorrow is only a vision,
> But today well-lived makes
> Every yesterday a dream of happiness

And every tomorrow a vision of hope.

Look well therefore to this day! Such is the salutation of the dawn.

The boy would awake every morning excited with the promise that he should look forward to "the bliss of growth, the glory of action and the splendour of beauty". That would be enough. He already exhibited a burgeoning excitement at the thought of an exploding kaleidoscope of possibilities of the future. What could be more exciting? Then, one amazing night, this unheralded event skyrockets him into a new dimension. No one had warned him of its imminent possibility, of the intensity and arousal of every cell of his body. What was that? It was exotic and mystical at the same time. He realised he had passed into new territory, but it was a secret too large to share. Who could he ask or tell? Certainly not his mother, or father, or siblings, or schoolmates.

It doesn't take long for him to realise he can reproduce this cataclysmic experience himself and thus begins a secret lifetime fascination with his ability to pleasure himself, quietly and quickly. With every orgasmic sensation, there is a release of the pleasure hormones, serotonin, dopamine and oxytocin. This increases the continuing need for repeat performances setting up a highly addictive trait for a "quick fix". Some researchers report that men masturbate sixty-five per cent more than women, men self-pleasuring 155 times a year and women for fifty-four.

The boy continues to learn more about reasons for this event, including sexual relations. He learns this from the great educator and leveller, sport, and the older boys in the sporting or football change rooms. At this stage, he will have learned very little from his father, school or church; his mother may have made a few obtuse offerings.

As philosopher Sam Keen states, a pecking order has been established in these hallowed men's caves. The alpha males are the ones who lead the conversation and it is invariably about sex. They want to be seen as the biggest and the best. They often display the swaggering, braggart personalities who build their reputation on sexual conquest, focussing on quantity, not quality. How many girls they can acquire and how many times they can "do" it – notches on the gun handle. The talk revolves around skiting how strong and "ripping" they were during sex, not around the fact they might have pleasured their partner. Instead of intimacy, sex for these boys was about masculine status and control.

Here the boy acquires by osmosis tips on how to meet and talk to girls, along with various information on how and where to have sex with them. But nothing about actually making love to them or loving them. The words respect and consent are never mentioned. Further down the order are the silent lovers, the ones who respect and love their partner, but say nothing so the boy learns little from them. Except at club functions where their respectful actions towards their partner are observed by the boy. He is learning from this also. As boys grow, most of them grow out of this change-room mentality. They make better judgements. However, some don't but stay in this model forever.

This old model needs to be thrown away, where ejaculation is always the quick end goal. It would be helpful that the man should start to embrace a model of partnered sex that focuses on pleasure, intimacy, connection and fun.

Women universally rate the overall relationship, in terms of warmth, caring, touching and closeness, as being as important as, if not more so, than erectile function. Note that we are talking sexuality here, not sex.

Sexuality relates to being male (or female – or any gender identity) and is independent of the ability to have penetrative sex. It may be useful to understand that the essence of what makes a good man has never changed: trustworthiness, a fierce capacity for love, unselfish action for the common good and the ability to laugh in the face of hardship – with no mention of sex. That is, humour, decency and joie de vivre.

At this stage of your personal journey and you may be ready to reveal your *homo* Moderna. You will now hopefully be aware you have acquired a more balanced playing field between partners. You may have acknowledged some masculine guilt concerning the creating of modern corporate, industrial, warfare and technological systems and noted the potential for these to dehumanise individuals, to create pollution and to generate destruction. You may also have become aware of the impact of the powerful influence of your mother and other authoritative women in your early life and also considered the magnetism and mystery of the alluring woman.

You may also realise the burden of these observations are not simply a male responsibility. These systems can only be created and perpetuated by consensual interaction between men and women, particularly of the elite, powerful, privileged and ruling classes. Within these structures, both genders maintain a high quality of life.

We might accept some guilt because men started and fought in wars (most of them unnecessary), and because we created technologies that proved to be addictive and polluting, but we are also aware that the women we married or partnered encouraged us to succeed and provide. This was also why men became excluded from their children, leaving this aspect to women– surely a great shame, albeit unavoidable in much of the past.

There can be no question but that the historical humiliation of women, the demeaning, the cruelty reported, are facts. But man's suffering from gender roles is also a fact.

We should now realise that the fastest path to ending the blame game is a committed relationship in which two people compassionately agree to work together to change the system.

Marriage/partnerships in most of the Western world start with the sentimental notion of romance. This is the initial powerful chemical and emotional reaction which always has the potential to end with authentic love. This is a period of unbroken intimacy, of passion, an enchanted world where a couple can be swept away for a period of time, where egos dissolve amid waves of pleasure, both or either partner giving in to the immediate need for the common cause. This spell, the honeymoon period, may last for days, weeks, years or sometimes can be intermingled with the fairy-tale ending, "forever". However, it takes more than a heart-fluttering romance to make a union last. Given the divorce rate, which is more than forty per cent in much of the world, love (lust), it turns out, is not enough. For genuine love to flourish, realities of children, money, religion, careers and many other issues will eventually direct them to enter into a respectful struggle, rejoicing in interdependence.

When there is a storm at sea, personalities can clash. To quote the writer William Arthur Ward: 'The pessimist will complain about the wind, the optimist expects it to change, but with reality, after debate, they agree to adjust the sails.' Instead of focussing on passive behaviour such as prolonged rumination on the negative, or impractical expectations of a miracle, adjusting the sails provides some sense of control.

True love is where two friends pledge to adjust the sails, to promise loyalty in working towards a compatible and agreed synthesis. They will vow to defend their separate integrities while respecting the other's integrity. They will meet only as equals, and will not cower or condescend.

Authentic love establishes there should be no boundary disputes. As Carl Jung has stated, where there is a power struggle, and one is dominant, love cannot exist. Their covenant will be to love one another justly and powerfully and while creating unassailable and sacred boundaries, they will respect their separate sanctuaries. Each will need his or her own time, space and areas of enshrinement.

With committed and regular conversation, they will move from solo to enter fully into mature love. Relationships, simply, are based on strong communication. Conversation will centre around topics such as a shared vision and aligned values.

Even before moving into a committed relationship, marriage or not, each will need to ask some tough questions of the other. Such as, what are your philosophies for handling debt? And finances? How will you split the bill? Thoughts on sickness and death, terminal illnesses. "Do not resuscitate" orders etc. Household chores – who does what? Stereotypes don't work anymore. How do you deal with different races, cultures, countries and religions? Children? How many? And who will be the main breadwinner? Are both in the couple happy with pets? Or not? How will you handle infertility? And infidelity? Divorce? What steps are you willing to take to prevent divorce? Schools – or not, universities for children? All big decisions that need to be thought about and discussed.

Ultimately, a strong relationship will only work if both partners display qualities of loyalty, reliability and dependability.

I am reminded of the certitude of the Irish poet and writer, John O'Donohue. He impresses we should search for an *anam cara*, literally, a soul-mate.

With this *anam cara*, you could share your most intimate thoughts, your innermost self, your mind and your heart. In this love, you are understood as you are without mask or pretension.

As a twenty-two-year-old, I didn't consider my life was too different from the experience and standards of males of my era, relevant to the 1960s. I was never an alpha male, as revealed at boarding school. My masters and peers found absolutely no leadership qualities in me at all. I did not attain the status of a prefect or captain of anything.

I thought this would bother me, but strangely it didn't. I was very comfortable and aware of who I was at this stage of my life – and of my potential. I was a work in progress. My life was just beginning. I had seen leadership at work and took silent note. I would find out later if it was important to lead. There are many ways to do this. But first I would need to work on my strengths and, if necessary, lead from within.

Being a fourth-generation Australian farmer, I looked forward to going back to the farm after school. That was my only plan. However, I was about to learn an important life-lesson on the delusions of control. The universe can reverse everything in a flicker. With only a few weeks to go to finish my school year, I received a letter from my father informing me he had sold the farm. I had no plan B!

We moved to Brisbane. I tried many jobs until I settled in the Public Service. And I certainly played sport, athletics, boxing and rugby as well as richly experiencing the customary youthful rites of passage in my social life. I finally attended university and it was here, in my second year of studying physiotherapy, my life was about to pivot wildly.

I was invited to attend a twenty-first birthday party of a former girlfriend. When I arrived, her house was buzzing, being full of university students. As I was looking from the veranda into the living room, it happened – just as the romance novels proclaimed. I glimpsed her face, her beautiful face, across a crowded room. In that instant, astoundingly, I felt the effect of an explosion of pheromones flooding my bloodstream. Oxytocin, dopamine and other feel-good chemicals jarred into place like a velvet-edged, exhilarating bear trap, triggering in me an exciting, sudden, deep yearning. Enchanted, I watched her walk across the room and sit down. This mysterious attraction compelled me to believe that I must get to know her.

As nobody was next to her, I conjured up courage to walk up and sit beside her. She flashed a disarming smile – one she still uses to break down the inner defences of censurers. For me, it was over. The evening went by in a blur, but by the time I had driven home that night, I had committed myself to courting and marrying this vision.

I have no doubt that then, and now, this is how "love", in its purest sense, may begin.

The best advice my wife and I received before our marriage

came from a marriage counsellor. We committed to attend a series of six presentations called "pre-*cana* talks", which were effectively designed to prepare couples for marriage. One counsellor advised us to have a "cocktail hour", every evening. No matter how late or tired, it is worthwhile for both partners to discuss the day's events, honestly and openly. This way we could appreciate how the day's events may have influenced either of us. Critically, any differences of opinion or conflicts could be discussed, any cracks patched as they develop.

I am very aware that every individual and every relationship is different and can be fraught with many unpredictable twists and turns, including luck, however, after fifty-seven years of marriage, this ritual still serves us well. I am still enchanted.

Millennials – Generation Y (1981-1996 – those now approaching forty years old) – see marriage and relationships a bit differently. Psychiatrist and relationship specialist Dr George West reports this demographic are two generations into a divorce-ready culture. Everyone they know has been touched by divorce at some level and they don't buy this idea that you meet someone, start a relationship and have a "happy ever after".

West continues, 'Millennials more readily access information and question the quality of the information they obtain. This generation is changing our culture at a fundamental level. When it comes to relationships, I believe it will be for the better.

It is an exciting possibility that the present generation of 'about-to-become parents' could be more open to preventing divorce than any generation before them.'

Ultimately, we have to remind ourselves that, in partnerships (of any defined gender) we are in this together, completely equal with every human right. We've had a long history together. We have to appreciate elements of our life began 3.8 billion years ago. We have been given one sliver of this time to savour. Our species, *Homo* sapiens, are the victorious result of many variations and random mutations wrenched from our early ancestors who first stood erect two million years ago. As males, we can still relate to our direct *Homo* sapiens hunter-gatherer forefathers, and can still be influenced by the chivalrous crusader knights. We can also see ourselves as Chris, the contemporary man in the introduction to this book.

But we are different from them – we have evolved to be much more than these men. We have the opportunity to throw off the shackles of these bastions of masculinity, to escape from our ivory tower of manhood, of machoism. We can now put out our hand and share equally again with our natural binary partners (or any other partner) unconditionally supporting each other and sharing our unique views of the world.

We can now imagine a world where gender does not define a person any more than race or ethnicity does. On that note, concerning race, as African-American actor Morgan Freeman comments, 'If we would recognise that there is only one human race and stop talking about races", we would come to realise skin colour is due to nothing more than the different environments our distant ancestors found themselves in.'

I would add this reasoning is also the case for different ethnicities.

For myself, I have found my DNA heritage consists of many ethnicities, Irish, Scottish, Welsh, Vikings (Scandinavian), Baltic, Iberian, Ashkenazi Jewish and Italian and I am Australian. Surely, this evidence of a global cocktail must also help to imagine a better world.

Finally, I would suggest that a life partner has much to recommend. One who you can commit to unconditionally and fully. This type of relationship creates a host of practical benefits including support for helping you to follow a dream, and vice-versa. There are also cardiovascular benefits, as the relationship is established, endorphins and hormones oxytocin and vasopressin create 'an overall sense of wellbeing and security which leads to lower blood pressure and heart rate,' as suggested by researchers at Chicago's Loyala University.

Also, a UCLA study found married couples live longer than their single counterparts. Another study from Harvard backs this up.

The Harvard study of adult development is one of the world's longest studies of adult life, health and happiness. More than eighty years ago, researchers at Harvard enlisted hundreds of participants who agreed to a wide range of interviews, questionnaires, physicals and extensive physiological measurements. The study began in 1938 with 268 men who were sophomores (second year university student) at Harvard between 1938 and 1944. (Of significance to this book, the participants were all males. Women weren't in the original study because the college was all male).

The researchers have since collected a cornucopia of data on their physical and mental health.

Of the original cohort recruited, as of 2017, only nineteen were still alive, all in their mid-nineties. (One of the original recruits was President John F Kennedy).

Over the years, researchers have studied the participants' health trajectories and their broader lives, including their triumphs and failures in careers and marriages. The findings have produced startling lessons:

> Our relationships and how happy we are in our relationships has a powerful influence on our health. Close relationships, more than money or fame, are what keep people happy throughout their lives. Those ties protect people from life's discontents, help to delay mental and physical decline, and are better predictors of long and happy lives than social class, IQ or even genes. Several of these studies found that people's level of satisfaction with their relationships at age 50 was a better predictor of physical health than their cholesterol levels were. The people who were most satisfied in their relationships at age 50 were the healthiest at age 80.
>
> The researchers also found that marital satisfaction has a protective effect on people's mental health. They found that people who had happy marriages in their 80's reported that their moods didn't suffer even on the days when they had more physical pain. Those who had unhappy marriages felt both more emotional and physical pain.
>
> The study also found that loneliness kills, confirming the evidence already discussed. Humans are social creatures. We thrive through connections to those around us. Those who felt isolated were less happy and experienced notably earlier deterioration in mental and physical health than others. Loneliness has just as large a

negative impact on our health as smoking or alcoholism. While we would embrace solitude, the quality and depth of our social connection is critical to our wellbeing.

Quality over quantity. The researchers found that the quality of relationships was more impactful on health and happiness than the quantity of relationships. A few deep bonds are worth more than hundreds of weak ones.

The Harvard researchers concluded that as ageing starts at birth, people should start taking care of themselves at every stage of life. After all, ageing is a continuous process.

I feel that it is judicious to start by taking care of yourself and your relationship early in life and set yourself on a better course for ageing. The best advice I have found is: 'Take care of your body as though you were going to need it for a hundred years – because you might.'

The loving feather is a gift – it is one you have to work at. True love fosters a connection that goes beyond the superficial. It is a bond that involves building relationships, understanding each other's core values and beliefs and gaining perspective on the other's physical, emotional and intellectual life goals. It involves listening to your partner's intimate disclosures in a supportive, patient and non-judgmental fashion.

CHAPTER NINETEEN

The Wild Feather – Go Wild

Security is mostly a superstition,
It does not exist in nature,
Nor do the children of men
As a whole experience it.
Avoiding danger is no safer
In the long run than outright exposure,
Life is either a daring adventure or nothing
– **Helen Keller**

'In wildness is the preservation of the world,'
– **Henry David Thoreau (1817-1862)**

Our mental and physical health cannot be understood simply in the narrow context of urbanisation and by the constructs and confinements of the modern social world. Scratch under our skin and you will find a primitive being yearning for wildness, for a primal connection to raw nature. He will be searching for access to vistas which satiate his DNA, mountains, tundras, bushlands, rivers, deserts, animals, birds and flora of every kind. To be healthy, we have to include the relationship of humans to other species and ecosystems.

These connections have a deep evolutionary history; they have profound psychic significance in the present time. Our spirits need to soar beyond the panorama of cement canyons and steel and glass cathedrals and buildings. We need to escape to wild, open places where we can again reignite our survival skills and exist in an environment not fabricated by humans.

There is a basic need to stimulate our slumbering instincts and senses, to feel our physical strength and the vigour of effort. Even to sit and gaze at wide vistas, oceans, mountains and meadows settles the heart and connects us to an existence and time when men had a rare feeling of truly being a man.

Industrialisation, domestication and urbanisation tend to diminish our perspective of our own importance. We seem to lose relevance, to be average, a number in a system, expendable. Wildness changes this and we suddenly become aware of ourselves.

A 2020 study by the University of Washington identified elements important for city-dwellers searching for a meaningful interaction with nature. The answers included encountering wildlife, walking along the edge of water, gazing out at a view, or following an established walking trail. Trails offer an antidote to our post-industrialised complacency and materialism.

David Strayer, a cognitive psychologist at the University of Utah has demonstrated that participants in a three-day wilderness backpacking trip not only feel restored, but their mental performance also improves.

On the third day, Strayer reported, being in nature allowed the prefrontal cortex, the brain's command centre, to dial down and rest. The senses recalibrate and participants could smell things and hear things they couldn't before.

This concept was also an intuition through history. Parcellus, the 16th century German-Swiss physician, wrote: 'The art of healing comes from nature, not from the physician.'

In 1798, sitting on the banks of the River Wye, poet William Wordsworth, marvelled at how 'an eye made quiet by the power of harmony,' offered relief from 'the fever of the world.'

I have regularly experienced this sensation, particularly after wilderness visits to outback Australia, and to great rivers, mountains and jungles of the world, but none more so than in Africa. Especially while enjoying game park drives, jungle walks and one very memorable safari canoeing down the Zambesi. On this adventure I encountered intermittent episodes of raw fear, but mainly a sense of freedom during long periods of tranquillity from being in harmony with nature.

The Zambesi River starts in the highlands of Angola and forms the borders of several countries on its way to the ocean. It is the fourth largest river in the world and generates great power. This power is manifest in the awe-inspiring Victoria Falls, one of the supreme sights on the planet, as the 1700-metre-wide river dives in five cataracts into a 108-metre chasm.

My wife and I began our adventure by flying into Lake Kariba at the headwaters where the Zambesi had been dammed. Here we met our armed guide and our six fellow canoeists (two in each canoe). We endured an unexpected and nervous three-kilometre walk through lion country to where our canoes had been prepared. We were given a safety talk, learning that more people are killed by hippopotami than by any other animal in Africa (one a day), and how to deal with any other animals we might encounter in the game parks, including the crocodiles which line the river banks. We were told what to do if we tipped over or were attacked

– during potential encounters with Zambian border patrols.

The fully loaded canoes appeared reasonably stable. Which was just as well as one of the most dangerous sections of the river was at the beginning. Here the headwaters formed rapids, back currents and whirlpools as it raced through a magnificent gorge carved for itself over aeons.

It was a rude challenge to suddenly acquire and sharpen paddling and canoeing skills. However, I was strongly motivated by sighting myriad crocodiles lining the banks, then silently slithering into the water as we encroached on their territory. After a couple of hours of intense struggling, the waters settled and our adrenalin also settled. Then it became rather pleasant simply allowing the five kilometre-an-hour current to transport us.

It was a chance to recover and appreciate the truly wild scenery and isolated area around us. We ate a nervous lunch on the banks of the river in the game park, always with one eye on the surrounding bush and the other on our gun-toting guide, making sure he didn't stray too far from us.

This was the pattern at all mealtimes, although after we'd relearned some animal behaviour and sharpened our dormant primitive survival skills, our breaks ashore became a rewarding natural adventure.

We spent our first night camped on an island in the middle of the river. Our neighbours were a fat crocodile lazing on the opposite bank, its iridescent, beady eyes focussing on us, and a large family of hippos who conducted a noisy midstream serenade all night. To this cacophony, the occasional distant lion roar, leopard cough or hyena laugh increased our uneasiness that we were sleeping in a natural zoo with no bars.

When dusk settled, events began to happen outside our campfire's circle of light, reaching us as muffled disturbances. Then muzzled screams raised a prickling of hair with an unease that stretched back to our own species' genesis. As the light faded, a magical event occurred as first one, then two, and then hundreds of brilliant fireflies illuminated the darkening sky. They were backed by a blazing concert of sparkling, shimmering stars, burning and dazzling in the crystal air.

As I awoke early next morning, I was suddenly aware in the predawn half-light that my space was shared with two large elephants moving less than seven metres away. I shot a glance over to our guide and saw he had the situation well in hand, ready with his gun if the elephants panicked. Mercifully, they walked past us into the water and over the stream where they berated a hyena on the far bank. The trumpeting and screaming echoed down the valley in the still morning air as the rest of our camp awoke in shock.

As the trip continued, our knowledgeable guide was a storehouse of information about the river and animal behaviour, sharing stories wrapped in our collective human experience. There were indeed many instances which gave us time for story-telling and for personal reflection.

There were often long periods of silence as the monotonous splish-splash of the oars reinforced a powerful meditative sensation. Just as suddenly, our ruminations could be shattered when an irritated hippo reared its head and shoulders above the water, eyes round in outrage, made a sound somewhere between the roar of a steam engine and the snarl of a motor mower and charged towards our canoes. At that moment, his challenge was a raiser of hair and a merchant of adrenalin. Some sounds go right to the core of masculinity and survival.

At the end of these types of adventures, I had never felt more alive, never more in touch with my instincts. All my survivor senses sharpened and I was very much aware of the raw hunter crouching restlessly inside.

This mindfulness was particularly evident when climbing in the wilderness. This connection was first really discovered for me when I walked the Kokoda Track. Then I tackled and reached the summit of Mt Kilimanjaro at the age of sixty.

This was a triumph and satisfied me for some years. However, I realised my attachment to wilderness had allowed me to view life from a larger perspective. I would live life passionately; I would climb another mountain, higher than Kilimanjaro.

In December 2009, at age sixty-six, I began climbing Mount Aconcagua. At almost 7000 metres, it soars out of the Andes in Argentina, the highest peak outside the Himalayas. After eight days, we became trapped by a blizzard fifteen hundred metres below the summit. We were three weeks into a climbing season marked by terrible storms.

While here, I was subject to an interesting phenomenon. We were advised not to go outside at night to urinate; the freezing conditions were too cold at minus 30 degrees. The correct technique is to kneel inside the tent and use a container. We had two containers each, a blue one for drinking water and a green one for urination. Being green-blue colour blind wasn't helpful; I didn't feel confident of doing this, so I elected to brave the elements outside.

Expecting the scene to be bitter and black, I was shocked to see the landscape flooded with burning, silver light. The heavens were crystal clear. The stars and moon were so close and unhindered by atmosphere, they totally blazed. The Southern Cross was on fire right above me. In an intense physical and emotional experience, amounting to an epiphany, I was overwhelmed by a sudden and pleasing revelation that I was in union with the universe. I could reach out and touch the stars and their trillions of atoms would be the same as mine. The feeling of inclusion has never left me.

Some years later, while holidaying with my family at Currumbin on Australia's Gold Coast, I experienced a similar incident reinforcing Nature's ability to reconnect us to our inner primitive animus. The day was large, the scene idyllic and the sky and sea endlessly blue. The roaring surf was inviting as the morning sun pierced through the cresting waves, rendering them a translucent green. The crashing foam raced up the wide, beautiful beach. I hit the waves as quickly as possible.

While swimming outside the breakers, waiting for a set of a rollers to take me in, up twenty-two kilometres to the north along the beach, I could see Surfers Paradise floating as if in a mirage in the crystal air. Seven kilometres to the south Coolangatta was clear as a bell. I could see my family, children, grandchildren and extended family happily playing on the beach. I floated on my back, looking up at the limitless, deep indigo sky and once again was deluged by the strong emotions of deep tranquillity and universal connection.

It is tempting to denote some relevance to this experience, but I suspect psychologists would consider it an extreme mindfulness or meditative phenomenon, focussing and connecting the mind and psyche to the present.

Chapter Nineteen The Wild Feather – Go Wild

A couple of years later, in 2014, at seventy-one years, I was keen to be challenged by climbing in the wilderness again. This time, I would venture to the Caucasus mountains in Russia.

My earliest experience of the Caucasus came from my Grade 8 school reader – a story from mythology. I have a vivid memory of a macabre drawing of Prometheus, a Titan, the cousin of Zeus, being bound strongly to a rock – in the Caucasus. A vulture was devouring his liver which would eternally regrow as it was eaten, propelling Prometheus to a life of suffering. He had displeased Zeus by showing humans how to utilise fire. His agony became a universal symbol for creating triumph out of adversity.

I was hoping for some of Prometheus's strength. I aimed to climb Mount Elbrus, at 5642 metres the highest mountain in Europe.

Just travelling to the Caucasus was an adventure. After meeting my expedition leader, Mike, who happened to be a New Zealand physiotherapist, and team in Moscow, we flew for three hours deep into Russia. We landed at Mineralny Vody (mineral waters) an industrial town between the Black Sea and the Caspian Sea.

From here, we were driven in a minibus for three hours to our base in the rugged mountainous regions of the Baksan Valley in the Caucasus. Here we met our first Russian guide, Oleg, who reinforced the validity of the Prometheus myth. To my surprise, he volunteered that the rock Prometheus was alleged to have been bound to was indeed Mt Elbrus. Marvellous: In this aspect, my experience of life had done a full cycle.

For the next two days we set off on acclimatisation hikes. We tackled surrounding peaks around the base of Mt Elbrus, climbing higher each day. We then packed all our gear and moved by cable car and chairlift to the head of the valley and bunked in Barrels Hut at 3900 metres.

In the meantime, we received disturbing news that three days previously a Russian man and his wife had reached the summit of the lesser cone of Elbrus. While posing for a photo with both hands and metal walking poles raised high in victory, a sudden lightning strike flashed from the heavens to the poles, instantly earthing through the man. He died tragically celebrating his moment of triumph. His wife dug a hole in the snow and stayed with him all night.

Zeus, the keeper of the weather, was still around, amusing himself and randomly reminding us humans we were now in his territory.

After a few days of heavy workouts in the snow at about 4800 metres, summit day had arrived. We woke at 1 am, packed and dressed in our warmest high-altitude gear. We had breakfast at 2 am and then hit the snowfields at 3 am for the climb of Elbrus' west summit of 5642 metres. It was now seriously cold, minus fifteen degrees, and a slight wind added to the chill factor. It was a brilliant, clear night. Brushstrokes of snow streaked the ground.

At 5100 metres, above the ski and snowboarding fields, we tackled deep snow along steep 60 degrees slopes and ascended along a traverse across the volcano face. We were aiming for Elbrus Pass, the Saddle, between east and west summits of Elbus. This was extremely difficult and, indeed, rather dangerous. The exercise required strong use of crampons. It was dark and my headlight illuminated the very narrow snow path, confirming that one wrong slip could send me hurtling down the icy, snowy mountainside for hundreds or even thousands of feet.

At about 6 am, as the sun began to rise, a fleeting glance of the surrounding vista revealed a magical, staggering, rugged snow-covered mountain landscape down below, achingly beautiful to my eyes. Flickering lights from the darkened valleys emphasised dozing villages. It also revealed a steady stream of headlights following us up the same path as more climbers methodically hammered towards the summit.

Then, chillingly, even though the night was cloudless and the stars fairly blazed above, below me I noticed 'dry' lightning flashes crashing on to the base of the volcano, an eerie and unusual phenomenon. Zeus was out tonight and launching warnings. I quietly made a note not to raise my poles above my head, particularly if in victory.

The pressure was unrelenting; I found it difficult forcing a path through the fluffy snow. By 8 am I had become extremely exhausted. I forced myself to reach the saddle at 5350 metres, less than 300 metres from the top, still an hour and a half climb away but higher than any other mountain in Europe – the Matterhorn, Mont Blanc and the Eiger.

I had stumbled several times and I was aware that I was beginning to hallucinate. I would momentarily close my eyes, my brain grasping for sleep and I would visualise unfamiliar images. I intuitively understood this was serious. It is a sign of HACE (high altitude cerebral oedema). Our very experienced second guide, also named Oleg, insisted I turn around. In sixteen years of guiding he knew of only two other seventy-year olds who had reached this point. Team leader Mike also agreed I should stop. This would have to be close enough.

There is a point when the body screams "enough" but the mind can take over and push further. I was aware I had very little in the tank at that moment. If I heroically trudged on, I reasoned the effort could be dangerous. HACE can alter perception, often leading to euphoric and poor judgements. Even if I did manage to get higher, I would certainly have trouble descending.

As it was, coming down was dangerous and extremely difficult. My legs were like jelly, my quads collapsing. Oleg fastened a rope between us and steadily assisted me down the same treacherous pathway. I fell several times, but the rope and his strong hands stopped me sliding away. Realising the seriousness of the situation, he phoned below for a snowmobile to meet me at the 5100 metre mark, the upper end of the snowfields.

This turned out to be an unexpected upside in terms of excitement. The machine was driven by a character who would have fitted the mould of a fearless, cocky fighter pilot. I was grateful for his help but didn't expect the extent of the thrill to come. I sat behind him, braced my weakened thighs with my feet locked into the runner and numbly held on to bars behind me. He nudged the snowmobile over the rim of the ledge. My heart leapt. It faced a 1300 metre, sixty degrees straight down descent.

He accelerated and I gasped, barely muffling an expletive. The machine dropped away, flashing down the mountainside. Within a few seconds, I was intoxicated by the speed – dopamine and adrenalin racing through my body. No seatbelts, no metal protection, simply the rapture of freedom, motion and thunderous speed. Exhilarating. Not for a moment did he ease back on the throttle. We reached 85 km/h, the driver skilfully manoeuvring and zipping around other wide-eyed climbers and snowboarders who suddenly appeared in his vision. I was barely mindful that if he merely tapped an unseen rock or hard snow, the machine could career out of control with the two of us spinning wildly in different directions.

My already exhausted thighs were burning as I tried to push my feet further into the runners to stop sliding off the seat. My shoulders ached from fighting with the bars yet I didn't want the moment to stop. It was addictive and euphoric. Eventually, the driver spun to a halt at the bottom of the snowfield – suddenly releasing the tension. We were both laughing helplessly, reacting to the thrill of the moment. We had no common language, only the universal literacy of two boys enjoying the unadulterated rush of speed and danger.

In that moment, I could relate a little to the emotions expressed by Lighthorseman WC as he charged at breakneck speed towards the entrenched Turkish lines at Beersheba. Even though I wasn't being shot at, the intensity and exhilaration were such that I knew the memories would stay with me, searing to a high that I would probably never experience again.

Along these lines, it would be remiss not to include snorkelling and scuba diving as positive incursions into the wild.

I experienced my first scuba dive fifty years ago at Lady Elliott Island, a beautiful coral cay on the Great Barrier Reef. I still recall the excitement of witnessing a turtle swim through a coral arch in a brilliant coral garden. I was hooked from day one.

Whether exploring shipwrecks, swimming with ocean animals or simply taking in the sights on a coral reef, there are countless treasures waiting to be discovered under the waves. Diving encourages you to live in the moment, forcing all your senses into primordial viability.

It encourages long, deep breaths, the key to relaxation, but there is a special connection to the wild as you become immersed in a natural world far from your normal environment. I have sought these encounters all around the world.

I relished visiting the Solomons where I dived on wartime wrecks in Iron Bottom Sound; Espiritu Santo in Vanuatu, the setting for James Michener's *South Pacific* and loved diving here on the *President Coolidge*, a sunken troopship. Probably the prize was diving in Truk Lagoon in the Caroline Islands, in Micronesia, in the Western Pacific Ocean.

Truk was the island where the Japanese Imperial Army planned their notorious bombing missions on Pearl Harbor, Guam, the Philippines, Rabaul and Darwin.

Truk was undisputedly a diver's mecca. In February 1944, three US carrier task groups destroyed a massive sixty Japanese war vessels and two hundred war planes, all now resting on the bottom of the harbour. Because of their remoteness, they had rarely been visited or disturbed.

As I descended into the clear indigo water, a sunken destroyer came into clearer focus. While hovering over the bow, I was not prepared for the first visual impact. I found myself surrounded by a living, moving, brilliantly coloured ecosystem. Fascinating coral of all shapes, colours and sizes had overgrown the oppressive relics of war and sea life of all types had made their homes here. Beauty had overcome evil. The tragedy of war had created a magnificent kaleidoscope of artificial reef unmatched anywhere.

The wrecks had changed from barren, burnt hulks to repositories of new life. They acted as nurseries providing shelter for the breeding grounds of myriad fish life, from tiny iridescent blue coral fish to attracting predators such as barracuda and sharks to complete the food chain.

On the port side, a gaping torpedo hole showed where the vessel was sunk by an American Avenger torpedo bomber. I floated over other vessels revealing large impotent deck guns pointing to the surface, almost unrecognisable due to the marine growth on them. In the holds of one ship, I saw small arms, belted machine gun ammunition and 4.7 inch brass shell casings. In another hold were Zero fighter fuselages, wings and propellor blades.

Life and nature have triumphed in Truk Lagoon amid the scars and wreckage of war. Overgrown with a million forms of life, the evidence of man's folly in war will be completely absorbed in a few years by coral and history.

Research has shown that simply being in a natural environment reduces physiological markers of stress, including lowering blood pressure and the stress hormone cortisol. You don't need to challenge yourself physically to create a response. Nature offers a powerful form of mindfulness that supports calmer bodies and minds. Simply being there, allowing your eyes to gaze into the distance, is enough to make change.

CHAPTER TWENTY

The Healthy Feather

'A good laugh and a long sleep are the best cures in the doctor's book,'
– **Irish proverb.**

The initial motivation for me to write this book was to answer the question: 'Why don't men look after their health better?' At the outset, the journey took into account the historical context, then thrust this perspective forward to the present day. My observations were that very clearly we needed to change our destiny, which I proposed.

So there is a final component which I need to discuss, one which I consider to be important to living a meaningful and healthy life in this generation. It concerns accepting responsibility for your own health. There is endless advice from authorities, gurus, books, articles, television and media celebrities touting their programs and podcasts promising improved mental, physical, sexual and productive healthy lives. My advice is to take what you can from all these sources, but be highly selective and critical of most of them.

As part of transitioning to the future, allow me to suggest some personal insights. If we can add this feather, the healthy feather, to our pageantry, it will enhance every other feather. Our display will be brilliant.

Chapter Twenty The Healthy Feather

My first suggestion, as just mentioned, is to take responsibility for your own health. Do not delegate this authority or rely on other family members to monitor your health. Be prepared to share the decision-making and management, but you must be the alert, proactive and prophylactic proprietor. Be collaborative with your general practitioner and plan an annual check-up. Screen appropriately for disease prevention, check on cardiac and blood pressure, lungs and pulmonary efficiency by carrying out a benchmark stress test (MVO2) and lung capacity and functional tests. Screen for cancers, prostate, bowel, testicular, skin and other systemic diseases, diabetes etc, as well as hearing and eyesight. Carry out a full work-up on blood and urine annually. Monitor your weight and other healthy lifestyle factors.

Over the last fifty-seven years, as a sports and exercise physiotherapist, I have been privileged to treat a great many of my patients on a continuum. I have kept detailed records of their health from when they began their careers as younger athletes. I have documented them moving on to middle age with a different set of injuries, then to an ageing and gerontology demographic, with a different category of injuries and conditions, including prostate cancer and related side effects.

Recently, one of these long-term patients presented, I'll call him Bob, for me to assess his painful knee. He had been an elite rugby player in his youth, and now middle-aged at fifty years, he was clearly overweight. He had no recent significant history indicating why his knee may be painful, although his MRI showed serious arthritic changes to his patella and a complex, but non-displaced tear of the body and posterior horn of the medial meniscus.

I explained that meniscal tears and arthritic destruction were common for one in three men of his age group, and most were symptom free. I also gently pointed out that, he is over forty and biologically past his "use-by-date". Most of his joints would be degenerative but symptom-free. Documented evidence gives me the opportunity to add a caveat that if he exercises regularly most of his joints, muscles and tendons could remain symptom-free for many decades.

For his knee, I advised him the best line of treatment was to focus on losing weight, get generally fit and strengthen the quadriceps, the muscle group that supports, controls and stabilises his knee.

'How much do you weigh?' I asked provocatively.

'I am a few kilos overweight,' he smiled, 'probably about 85 kilograms.'

'How much were you at your fighting weight? This is your weight when you were at your fittest and in your prime, probably about twenty to twenty-four years of age.'

'Probably about seventy kilos,' he said, which agreed with my records.

I asked him to pick up a supermarket bag I kept in my gym. I told him it had some weights in it. He was surprised he could barely lift it.

'How much is in there?' he asked, perplexed.

'Ten kilograms,' I said. I then weighed him and found he actually weighed ninety kilos. I pointed out the extra twenty kilograms he was carrying was twice the amount in the supermarket bag. That extra weight was being carried every moment by his knees, back and feet. I even more gently explained he was not only overweight but his body mass index (BMI) was just over thirty. He was obese.

BMI estimates your total amount of fat. It is a person's weight divided by the square of their height.

Obesity is one of the great health problems of the 21st century. Being overweight can impact on almost everything you want to achieve in your life. Some of the co-morbidities related to overweight and obesity can be seriously life threatening. These include hypertension, stroke, coronary artery disease and congestive heart failure, cancers (breast, endometrial, ovarian, colorectal, oesophageal, kidney, pancreatic, prostate), type 2 diabetes, asthma, chronic back pain, osteoarthritis, pulmonary embolism, gall bladder disease and an increased risk of disability.

Studies have confirmed that obesity results in decreased life expectancy and can certainly impact on sexual health. Being overweight also can produce a regrettable stigma, discrimination and social bias, which can lead to certain mental disorders including low self-esteem, eating problems and motivational disorders. All these directly or indirectly affect quality of life.

'How do I lose weight?' asked Bob, whose age group sits smack in the middle of the "sandwich generation", the cadre dealing with pressure from either side, educating children, mortgages, work and being aware of caring for ageing parents.

I explained weight-loss programs appear in many guises. Fundamentally they aim to do the same thing, put less kilojoules into your body while you burn more up. There are many valid ways to do this, keeping in mind many dieting programs are gimmicks and promise the world.

The Butterfly Foundation (an institution catering for the needs of people with eating disorders – email support@butterfly.org.au), offers a stark warning – never go on a diet as it could be the first steps on the slippery slope to an eating disorder.

It warns that extreme fasting, eliminating food groups, excessive caloric restriction and skipping meals can all lead to disordered eating, a point which is the single most important indication of the onset of an eating disorder. This can also lead to health concerns such as depression, anxiety, nutritional and metabolic problems and weight gain.

As I warned Bob, 'Even when you do lose weight, evidence has shown after five years as many as ninety-five per cent of dieters will return to where they started and forty-one per cent will have regained more weight than they lost. The reality is you need to seriously commit to change your behaviour. And it is exercise that makes a plan stick. A diet alone has been found to be nowhere near as effective for fat loss as combining good nutrition with exercise.'

As researchers from *Men's Health* magazine state, as well as being beneficial in isolation, training (exercising) has proved to play a key role in diet adherence. Without introducing exercise and diet in harmony, you will have great trouble tipping the scales in your favour. Most of us underestimate the mental toughness required to resist cravings (fast food and sugar, fat, salt, ingredients which food companies often insert by stealth), but research shows that even small amounts of physical activity can strengthen willpower. Hitting the gym not only burns kilojoules; it also steels you against the desire, or addiction, of fast foods.

As creatures of habit in our eating routines, we tend to eat about the same amount at mealtimes. Emeritus Professor "Frank" Gardiner's suggestion of eating a morsel less at every meal until a consistent weight loss is evident, seems a good ploy.

If you're training hard, you have the opportunity to break from nutritional austerity with a cheat day. If you rely exclusively on managing food intake, or dieting, to lose weight there is no room for slip-ups as you can't burn off extra kilojoules without exercise. Exercise, workouts and training are what turns any attempt to lose weight into a sustainable lifestyle, rather than a short-lived dietary denial.

How much exercise? You should consult a professional for this advice. Everyone's needs will be different, but there are a few consistent principles. The American Heart Association recommends at least 150 minutes of heart-pumping physical activity a week. That amounts to thirty minutes a day over five days. It also advises you can gain more benefits by being active for more than that, at least one hour a day (300 minutes a week).

This advice is reinforced by some brilliant research coming out of the Cleveland Clinic. In the past, intensive regular exercise has been theorised to be potentially associated with harm to the body compared with moderate exercise. This new research has raised the bar exponentially. (Mandsager K, et al. JAMA Network Open 2018).

Cleveland Clinic used data collected over from 1991 to 2014 of patients who received an exercise treadmill test (fitness test). Some 122,000 patients young, middle age and older (average age 53.4 years; 59.2 per cent male), were evaluated representing 1.1 million person-years of observation. Death occurred on 13,637 patients over the course of the study. Death from any cause was found to be inversely correlated to how fit the patients were.

The highest levels of fitness were associated with the highest survival or longevity, and this included older patients (70 and 80+). There was no observed threshold in benefit.

The results scream loudly that fitness could be the greatest secret to longevity. Preliminary findings suggest that when it comes to exercise more is better with no known upper limit of benefit or threshold. In other words, the fitter you can become, the better. 'Never regret a workout,' thus seems a good mantra.

If you have done nothing for years, set a reachable goal for today, maybe five minutes walking. Anything is always better than nothing. As you adapt to one level, slowly overload. Increase intensity, distance, time, speed or resistance by about ten per cent. Any more than ten per cent and you run the risk of creating damage, straining soft tissue structures, ligaments etc. or just becoming plain exhausted, which can diminish motivation.

As you age, you may need to do more than the hour of exercise a day. With ageing, two main physiological problems can confound progress and maintenance. First metabolism slows by about two per cent a decade from age twenty-five. This relates to your basic metabolic rate, which is defined as the amount of energy it takes to maintain your muscle mass, your fat mass, your bones and all the activities of your organs. Basically, how much energy it takes to keep us alive.

This means as you get older, you may need to decrease the amount you eat by a corresponding amount in order to offset that metabolic change and to maintain your weight. Or you can monitor your physical activity by increasing it and doing extra exercise.

The second problem associated with ageing can be sarcopenia, which is loss of muscle mass and function. Physically inactive people can lose as much as three to five per cent of their muscle mass each decade after age thirty. So that by sixty you could have lost up to fifteen per cent of your muscle mass. Any loss of muscle matters because it lessens strength and mobility. Sarcopenia speeds up at about sixty-five and is a factor in frailty, increasing the likelihood of falls and fractures in adults. Even active people can lose a degree of muscle mass with ageing, so there is a strong call for increased resistance training as you get older. Basically, you should do weights or Pilates twice a week. Recent research suggests exercising in the morning is more effective at reducing belly fat and blood pressure. (Paul Arciero, Skidmore College, New York).

It is important to pigeon-hole your day, plan a routine in your diary and stick to it. Exercise, particularly strength training, has to be a priority. You do not need to lift heavy weights, but if you do it must be done with correct technique. You may need to begin with a tailored program with a personal trainer.

If you continue having trouble achieving weight loss you may need to consult a sports dietician, specialist physician or endocrinologist to look at other factors including maybe hormones or genes.

To make a viable and continuous assault on mid-section belly fat, put on your runners, gym clothes or swim togs. What is important is to work towards achieving a behaviour change leading to a lifestyle change. This means pledging to an admission that you need to change; then commit to a discipline that you will adhere to.

This concept is not easy in reality. Doctors say they are failing to cut through to overweight patients with the message that obesity can lead to major health problems, with very few patients prepared to do anything about it.

Australian Medical Association Queensland president Dr

Dilip Dhupelia said the overwhelming majority of its doctors said their advice was not being heeded and patients lacked the motivation to tackle their weight issues.

The latest figures show that sixty-six per cent of adults and twenty-five per cent of children in Queensland are overweight or obese. This compares with developed countries globally. In 2017-18, in Australia, three in four men were overweight or obese, while only fifty per cent were deemed physically active. Nearly ninety per cent of doctors said their patients were not prepared to change their diet or to exercise, even when they were aware of the health dangers of being overweight or obese.

'Clearly we are losing the battle of the bulge,' Dr Dhupelia said. 'We are very surprised general practitioners are seeing an increase in obesity rates and the apathy of patients who know what the risks of obesity are but are not prepared to do anything about it. We relate it to the easier availability of fast food, more time on activities that are sedentary, such as screen time and social media and less participation in sports and activities.'

To me, this is a national emergency, one that calls for a co-ordinated response from government, universities and business. In the meantime, for individuals, there may be a role for an experienced motivational coach, sports psychologist or exercise physiologist to get things moving.

While focussing in on exercise as a treatment and prevention, we should not ignore physical activity as part of work and general day-to-day living when we prescribe exercise. Exercise is a broad term and a subset of physical activity. In this context, exercise has the added element of being enjoyable through socialising, or as a hobby, a marvellous by-product.

'If we had a pill that conferred all the confirmed health benefits of exercise, would we not do everything possible to see that everyone had access to this wonder drug?' (Professor E Sallis, Fontana, CA).

Australia's Exercise is Medicine (EIM) initiative is part of a global campaign to increase physical activity. As well as exercise being a major influence on managing obesity, research shows there are many marvellous trade-offs. Regular exercise at the correct intensity can:

- Significantly improve overall health.
- Reduce the risk of heart disease by forty per cent. (Percentages do vary over time)
- Lower the risk of stroke by twenty-seven per cent.
- Reduce the incidence of diabetes by almost fifty per cent.
- Reduce mortality and risk of recurrent breast cancer by almost fifty per cent.
- Lower the risk of colon cancer by over sixty per cent.
- Decrease depression as effectively as medications or behaviour therapy.
- Reduce the risk of developing Alzheimer's disease by one third.

The online module and EIM resources can be accessed at www.exerciseismedicine.com.au

In light of the above mention of Alzheimer's disease and cognitive loss, this seems an appropriate moment to discuss hearing loss. When considering hearing loss from my own perspective, I suspect confronting this issue was one of the smartest feathers I added to my plumage.

Research has shown that men typically wait about ten years to address hearing loss after the first signs appear. New Australian research has revealed hearing aids may help prevent dementia and boost brain capacity as well as preserve hearing into old age.

A University of Melbourne study of almost a hundred senior citizens found almost all of them had significant improvement in their cognitive function after using a hearing aid for eighteen months. Associate Professor Julia Sarant said initial findings suggested hearing aids may make an enormous improvement in delaying dementia. The study found it can at least delay cognitive decline and potentially dementia.

After assessing the brain function and various other health indicators of ninety-nine people aged from sixty-two to eighty-two attending the university's audiology clinic, the researchers were able to show a clear link between the severity of a person's hearing loss and a decline in their cognitive function. However, when the team reassessed participants eighteen months after they were fitted with hearing aids 97.3 per cent had a clinically significant improvement or stability in "executive function", the pre-frontal cortex. This refers to the mental skills required to plan, organise information and initiate tasks that can be diluted with dementia.

They found that even for people with mild hearing decline, loss of cognitive function can be thirty to forty per cent faster than for a person with normal hearing. It is important to understand you actually hear with your brain, the ear is merely a conduit. If the conduit is damaged, the message does not reach your brain.

A report on risk factors for dementia in the prestigious *Lancet* journal (21 April 2018) stated that the single most important thing an individual can do and modify to prevent Alzheimer's is prevent hearing loss. This can reduce their chances by nine per cent. Other modifiable factors are smoking (five per cent), depression (four per cent), physical inactivity (three per cent), social isolation (two per cent), hypertension (two per cent) and obesity (one per cent).

Further, a 2021 research article by Glick and Sharma highlighted the amazing abilities of the brain and its capacity for change. They reported neuroplastic changes may occur across the human lifespan as a result of disease, injury, dysfunction and learning (adult neuroplasticity). Based on their findings, it appears that untreated hearing loss is associated with neural reorganisation and cognitive deficits.

Resisting our tendencies for male denial (or lack of awareness), it is critical to have a hearing test at the first sign of deafness, an event generally noticed by a partner.

I am forever grateful that my partner (wife), a speech pathologist, insisted I have a hearing test the minute I started to unreasonably turn the television sound up, and repetitively asked her to repeat what she said.

Besides wearing hearing aids, there are several ways to prevent damage to your hearing.

Exercise has been shown to reduce hearing loss. All exercise boosts circulation, which means more oxygen gets to the sensitive and delicate hair cells which bend and respond to vibrations from sound waves. Yoga is particularly helpful for protecting the ears because it has been proved to lower blood pressure as well as reduce symptoms of stress, both of which impact on how well you hear.

Being more than a most healthy weight can also affect a person's hearing, as can having diabetes. This is probably because abdominal fat leads to high blood pressure, causing stress in the body and vascular changes. Diabetes puts a load on the body and causes glucose to be stored as fat. So it pays you to keep your weight down and have a blood-glucose test arranged by your general practitioner.

Proceed with caution when using power tools, lawn mowers, outboard motors and chainsaws. Wear ear protection every time. Be careful with loud music, particularly using headphones and ear buds for more than two hours a day. It is not only domestic tools that damage inner ear hair cells. Be wary of home appliances, hairdryer, coffee grinder, vacuum cleaner, blender and Thermomix.

And quit smoking. This has been found to be associated with hearing loss.

Finally, it has been found that iron deficiency is also associated with hearing loss, so include leafy greens and folate, vegetables, nuts, lentils, whole wheat, brown rice and some red meat (the Mediterranean diet) in your meals.

But how do you plan for change?

An effective system that worked for me was to imagine how I would like my health to be in five years. I decided on this plan when I was thirty after my first MVO2 (stress test). I would set a goal by developing a proposal for my health and life, much like you would a business plan. Such a five-year plan will enable you to envisage what you want to look like, how fit, strong, responsive, independent and resilient you would want to be, as well as how healthy, physically and mentally, you would like to be.

Every morning, I recite this plan as a mantra and let it reinforce the message that to fulfil these requirements in five years' time, I do it every day forever. I plan each day, week and month and work at it as I would a business strategy. I have found if I exercise first thing in the morning it has the bonus and advantage of getting the 'chore' out of the way. It also releases endorphins thus allowing me to approach the rest of the day with enthusiasm.

Keep one thing in mind. We have no drugs to combat ageing, frailty, mobility impairment, poor balance, muscle weakness, fatigue, poor endurance, cognitive impairment, injurious falls, poor sleep quality and quantity and, most importantly, functional dependency.

Exercise can address all of these issues. It should be the most prescribed pill in the history of mankind.

This book is not about recommending personal diet and exercise programs. There are no magic pills, special foods or exercises that in isolation will promote longevity, health and wellbeing. So be wary of fads and snake oil miracle cures. The best advice is to consult a health professional, dietician, nutritionist or medical personnel to help you plan a personalised program. This will assist in supervising and motivating you for the best chance of achieving a healthy lifestyle and developing a happy, creative and fulfilling whole.

Having said that, I am going to offer some suggestions concerning diet and exercise which may help with your choices and direction. Generally, a heart healthy diet is a cancer healthy diet is a longevity diet. Some regions of the world have followed traditional diets and lifestyles that have produced the world's healthiest and longest-lived people.

Dan Buettner is still uncovering secrets of centenarians in regions he calls the blue zones, in reference to the colour places on a map of the world to denote where these people thrive. Places where there are no overweight or obese people.

Sardinia, in Italy, is home to the world's highest concentrations of male centenarians.

Before Buettner, Italian doctor Gianni Pes discovered this tendency with the Sardinian population and interviewed more than 300 centenarians. He believed that steep streets, (requiring intense regular activity performing daily duties), zeal for family, reverence for elders, a matriarchal culture in which women bear most of the family stress, and a simple traditional diet explains much of this longevity, particularly for males. Pes also found that the spouses of centenarians live longer than the siblings of centenarians, suggesting to him that a caring partner helping with diet and lifestyle may make a bigger difference than genes; longevity could be trained.

Buettner has also documented the lifestyles and diets of other similar areas that have produced the world's highest rates of centenarians – Nicoya in Costa Rica; the Greek island of Ikaria; Japan's Okinawa island; and a community of Seventh-day Adventists in Loma Linda, California.

Until the late 20th century their diets consisted almost entirely of minimally processed plant-based foods, mostly whole grains, greens, nuts, tubers and beans. Buettner documented these foods as the four pillars of every longevity diet on earth. People ate meat on average only five times a month. They drank mostly water, herbal teas, coffee and some wine (which Buettner says confirms the belief that moderate drinkers live longer than non-drinkers). Notably, they drank little or no cow's milk, although meat, fish and dairy could be consumed in low amounts. They had limited or zero consumption of refined sugar and other processed foods. The Loma Linda community was the only one completely vegan and had no alcohol. The other communities enjoyed a glass of mainly red wine.

As globalisation spreads, processed foods, animal products and fast foods are supplementing the traditional diets. Not surprisingly, chronic diseases are on the rise in the blue zones.

There were some other common ingredients of these communities. First, they had a cultural environment that reinforced healthy lifestyle habits, such as diet and exercise. They also encouraged strong social networks and did a great deal of gardening. They had developed a strong community spirit and seniors were valued as members of family and community. They fiercely resisted placing seniors in retirement villages and aged-care facilities.

- These communities also have extremely low-stress lifestyles. (The American Medical Association has noted that stress is the primary cause of more than sixty per cent of all human illness and disease). Over and above community and lifestyle factors being influential in longevity, there are many personal inner-life habits of people who live a long life. The Longevity Project (Hudson Street Press), the Landmark Eight-Decade Study by Friedman and Martin, reported some surprising discoveries. It found: The strongest predictor of long life was conscientiousness, which is synonymous with self-responsibility. Conscientious people were less likely to smoke, engage in risky behaviour and have accidents. They were more likely to focus on the big picture and make good health choices moment to moment.

- Avoiding stress alone does not add up to longevity, but being engaged with meaningful work does. A sense of purpose far outweighs the absence of hassles. Service to others ranked high in Friedman and Martin's study – even greater than feeling loved by others.

- Being part of something bigger than yourself: selfish

people die younger than people who belong to a group or movement. That can be a church, religion, social cause or healthy lifestyle. People who volunteer for something live longer than those who don't, but the 'something' has to be selfless. (Science shows that people who volunteer only for their own personal satisfaction live no longer than those who don't volunteer at all).
- Humming and singing. Yes, humming and singing. The healthiest people in the world seem to intuit the value of oxygen and regularly breathe deeply in some form or other. Rigorous daily exercise is one way; humming or singing, another.

Last, but not least, the authors found that centenarians laugh a lot. Reinforcing the concept that conscientiousness is an important personality trait to develop, research from Deakin University reveals that being conscientious and having an outgoing personality are the traits most closely linked to happiness, while neurotics and over-thinkers are least likely to be content.

The study provides the most comprehensive map of the links between personality traits and wellbeing ever compiled. Lead researcher Jeromy Anglim reported that finding bubbly extroverts were happy was not unexpected, but discovering conscientious people could be equally so was something of a surprise.

It was also a surprise to find modesty did not help people have a happy life. It was important to compare yourself favourably to others; being modest may have negative implications for wellbeing. This concept has been known since biblical times – 'Neither do men light a candle and put it under a bushel, but on a candlestick,' (Matthew 5.15). It is wiser to reveal your hidden talents – everybody may benefit.

Conscientiousness means someone who is organised, purposeful and disciplined. Someone who follows their conscience to do the right thing for a great or long-time good. Extroversion and conscientiousness are the strongest drivers of positive wellbeing.

There have been numerous diets promising weight loss, increased energy and so much more. Many fall into the fad category. They are popular for a minute but become obsolete the instant they prove to be ineffective and, in some cases, dangerous. They range from elimination plans to juice cleanses. The most recent popular ones are the 5:2 Diet, also known as the Fast Diet, the Keto diet, Paleo diet, Macrobiotic diet, Flexitarian diet, Weight Watchers and the Mind diet, but the largest trends in Australia at the moment would be vegetarian and vegan diets. These all have their place for different individuals and there are special programs for dieters working around gluten-free and specific food-intolerances.

However, although it has been around for quite a while, the diet deemed the best diet of 2019 by *US News and World Report* was the Mediterranean diet.. It is widely praised as one of the healthiest eating plans available. Inspired by the traditional eating principles of countries bordering the Mediterranean Sea, particularly Italy and Greece, and very like the longevity diets mentioned in the Blue-Zones earlier, it encourages the consumption of fruits, vegetables, fish and heart-healthy fats. Numerous studies have found it helps with weight loss, heart health, stroke prevention, diabetes prevention, and prevention of some cancers and premature death, and also deep sleep. It is particularly helpful for men diagnosed with prostate cancer, both in minimising the risk and in managing life after diagnosis.

Importantly, this diet boosts levels of the "good" bacteria in your gut. These in turn can produce a powerful anti-inflammatory agent as well as "feel good" chemicals that reduce anxiety. It can have a direct and immediate effect on hormone levels, mood, pain tolerance and energy levels, and is recommended to help desensitise persistent pain.

Most significantly, the Mediterranean diet has been shown to trump genetics in relation to cardiac health. A recent research article from Deakin University by Katherine Livingstone (lead author et al), has shown diet is the number one risk factor that we can influence in tackling heart disease, the leading cause of death in Australia.

Using a set of 300 genetic markers for cardiovascular disease and heart attack the Deakin team analysed the outcomes of 77,000 adults aged forty to sixty-nine, comparing their diet quality and genetic risk to their heart health over eight years. They found that people who had a high genetic risk significantly lowered their risk if they followed the Mediterranean diet.

Here is an example of a recommended Mediterranean diet:
- Emphasise fruits, dark green leafy vegetables, whole grains, legumes, lentils, pulses, beans, seeds, sunflowers, pumpkins.
- Snack on nuts, as they are a great source of protein and fibre; almonds, cashews, walnuts.
- Eat a rainbow of fruits and vegetables – orange, green, yellow, red, purple, white, eg grapes, apples, berries: strawberries, blueberries, raspberries, pears, carrots, broccoli, spinach, kale, garlic.

- Eat more fibre by switching to brown rice, quinoa, whole rye, lentils and beans.
- Choose low-glycaemic index (GI) carbohydrates – sweet potatoes, oats, wholegrain breads and wholegrain pasta. Cut back on high GI carbohydrates (white breads, cakes, donuts, sugars).
- A note on sugar, the recommended daily allowance is six teaspoons. Australians have as many as forty a day, often stealthily hidden in processed foods. Become a strong label reader of sugar content. Be aware that four grams of sugar equals one teaspoon. A 330 ml can of Coke contains 35 grams, about nine teaspoons, of sugar.
- Condiments: sea salt, pepper, turmeric, cinnamon.
- Essential fatty acids. Choose more omega 3 (anti-inflammatory) foods such as walnuts, flax seeds, salmon, tuna and mackerel, cherries, turmeric, dark green leafy vegetables, eggs and soy. Choose less omega 6 and 9 (pro-inflammatory) foods (margarine, chips, cookies, cakes, biscuits, salad dressings, chocolate bars). However, dark chocolate has natural antioxidant properties and has been shown to lower blood pressure – two squares after dinner, but only if it is seventy per cent cocoa.
- Olives.
- Resveratrol – found in skin of grapes, blueberries and raspberries, green tea. Have red wine with dinner (one or two glasses).
- Moderate use of full-fat yogurt (good source of probiotics) and low-fat cheese.
- Chicken.

- Eat less meat and dairy.
- Fish: salmon, sardines, mackerel, trout.
- Extra virgin olive oil.

If possible, all foods should be fresh, locally and organically grown.

Alcohol is the elephant in the room. It can damage your liver, brain, nervous system, heart and gut, among other things. The most accurate answers to how much alcohol is the right amount is no alcohol, as this is the healthiest option. The US Preventative Services Task Force recently updated its clinical guidelines for unhealthy alcohol use as follows:

Healthy adult men, aged 21-64 years, should not have more than four drinks a day or more than fourteen a week. Healthy men aged sixty-five or older should not have more than three drinks a day or more than seven a week, and

Healthy adult women of all ages should not take more than three drinks a day or more than seven drinks a week. A drink is considered as twelve ounces of beer, five ounces of wine or 1.5 ounces of liquor (spirits), which, of course, is impossible to find at a bar, hotel or restaurant. They often supply much more than that, often double.

Research is beginning to demonstrate that there is no safe level of alcohol. We are living during a historical obesity epidemic and alcohol is seven calories a gram (more than sugar which is four calories a gram, with four grams equal to one teaspoon). One of the problems with alcohol is not so much the carbs but that it tends to make you hungry. You are tricked into eating more while drinking and generally opt for salty, fatty foods which add kilograms to your body.

The other reason it helps to put on weight is due to the forever increasing measures and alcohol content in today's world. Beer was 3.2 per cent alcohol thirty years ago and now many beers are seven to ten per cent – more alcohol content and more calories an ounce. More than ever in human history.

Alcohol is now accepted as a true carcinogen that accelerates the risk of aggressive prostate cancer. Drinking alcohol in excess in the elderly also heightens the risk of falls, a potentially devastating outcome.

The good news uncovered by one landmark research project, particularly for older adults, is that those from this group who have a beer or wine each day appear to be protecting themselves from heart disease.

A Monash University-led study of 18,000 adults in their mid-seventies, reported in the November 2021 issue of the *European Journal of Preventive Cardiology*, found if these people drank five to ten standard drinks across the week, it gave them a significantly smaller chance of dying from any cause compared to teetotallers.

The adults, with an average age of seventy-four, were followed for four and a half years. Lead researcher Associate Professor Robyn Woods said previously the focus had only been on younger adults. She said, 'It's that range of five to ten standard drinks a week where we saw real benefit for reducing the mortality risk, and also on cardiovascular disease.'

In view of these disclosures, I probably won't quit my regular glass of red (in moderation, as in the Mediterranean diet) but I am watching the amount they sell me, and what I eat with it.

CHAPTER TWENTY-ONE

The Newly Adorned Dashing Peacock

'Life isn't about finding yourself, Life is about creating yourself,'
– George Bernard Shaw

The reader may be aware most of the preceding ideas for this book flowed from the mind of an octogenarian. I consider this to be an advantage and a privilege. I have lived through four of the most transforming generational cohorts in history, ones that bookended the twentieth century.

My father's generation, the Great Generation (born 1901-1927) lived through a significant depression in the 1930s, and survived the Second World War. These men were definitely master of the house and retained much of the creed of the crusaders. Some of their traits were:

- Personal responsibility – take the blame, play fair.
- Humility – modest and humble.
- Work Ethic – hard work enabled survival.
- Frugality – saving every penny and every scrap of food.
- Commitment – one job or one marriage most often lasted a lifetime. Integrity – value of honesty and trustworthy.

Some of the traits that distinguished them were handed down

to my generation – the baby boomers (born 1946-1964) – even though I was actually born in 1943 right on the cusp of the boomers.

The boomers retained certain of those characteristics but they came of age at a time of increasing affluence, leading to cultural changes and new social and sexual freedoms. This era coincided with the emergence of the Pill, a burgeoning feminist movement and a willingness to break out of the restrictions of earlier years. However, during this age of reform they rejected traditional values which seems to be a trade-off for this independence and confidence. There is a documented cognitive decline as they aged relative to older generations. Physical inactivity, depression, cardiac issues and diabetes are all implicated.

Fathers of this era, the 1950s, sixties and seventies generally had a tougher burden providing for their families, most being the sole providers and breadwinners, still fulfilling the stereotype of the generation. They often existed by stoicism, frequently having a poor relationship with their children.

Divorce laws were cruel and could confine a couple to existing in wretched marriages. Abuse and domestic violence were never discussed or even considered, as they were regarded as private and personal issues, further trapping individuals of either gender into fragile relationships. Gender roles were clear and there was little tolerance, legally or communally, for gender diversity of any kind.

My son's generation, Generation X (born 1965 to 1980) is unique because of its use of technology, video games etc and a strong work ethic. This cohort has been credited with entrepreneurial tendencies. There is a definite trend for more sharing of family duties and decision-making, particularly as women entered the workforce exponentially. Gen-Xers had watched the boomers turn into workaholics in a workforce that encouraged long hours and a hard grind. Researchers found Gen X professionals in mid-life instead sought a balance of work and life and introduced the idea into the workplace.

My grandson's generation, the millennials (born 1980 to 2000) are often termed digital natives and are marked by elevated use of the internet, mobile devices and social media. They are family-centric and team-orientated and revel in collaboration. They are tolerant to gender diversity, viewing gender as a psychological spectrum where gender exists on a continuum that can move fluidly between masculine and feminine.

They challenge the hierarchal status-quo, are ambitious, curious and driven by individuality. Technology and Covid have allowed women to work from home, further levelling the playing field for gender equity, although it has some distance to go. However, men continue to share family and home duties.

From my position I have observed a clear changing perspective of what it is that defines a male.

A great majority of young men now reject harmful masculine stereotypes, raising the prospect of new generations of men who may not be aggressive and may be more willing to seek help early. I see them comfortably fitting into the role of sharing equally with their partners.

Clearly the future for males is controlled by an emerging thoughtful male who has the strength and the insight to reject, to redefine and reimagine who we are and where we are going.

We may have some distance to go, but I like where the modern young man is going.

Chapter Twenty-One   The Newly Adorned Dashing Peacock

*

'How do I look now?' he asked, still preening in the mirror.
'Absolutely marvellous.'
'Do you like my new feathers?'
'I love them. They are beautiful.'
'And the dowdy ones?'
'They are all gone – you are very attractive now – absolutely dashing.' 'Hmmm. Would you like to see my etchings?'

But wait, there's more. I have included a bonus chapter – an expansion of the proposed relevance of the hunter gatherers to our story.

CHAPTER TWENTY-TWO

The Ancient Feather

'Civilisation began the first time an angry person cast a word instead of a rock,'
– **Sigmund Freud, neurologist.**

East Africa. The vast savannah. Late afternoon, one day 200,000 years ago. The young warrior, Baan, slowly and carefully stood to his full height. His eyes narrowed as they peered into the distance, over the tufts of tall elephant grass and through the familiar acacia and baobab trees. The sun, still hot, was lowering over the scene. He and his band of ten hunters were a little concerned – they had not yet sighted a suitable target, possibly an antelope or zebra.

Baan had a sleek, athletic body, nudging six feet (183 centimetres). His height and leanness were perfectly adapted for efficient heat dispersal; his shoulders were well muscled, sinewy and strong, his back tapering to a fine waist. He moved stealthily, his glistening back and powerful buttocks capable of quickly propelling him on fast, lean legs. His body was suitably acclimatised to running over these plains and, when necessary, moving around jungle entanglements.

He had black hair, coiled for ventilation and cropped at his shoulders. His skin was lustrous, ebony black and satin smooth.

His face was rugged with a strong jawline and perfect white teeth, shining behind large and full lips, designed to assist body heat dissipation. His nose was typically wide, ensuring a smooth air flow for efficient cooling and less humidification.

These ten men, the hunters, had developed into being Baan's closest friends as they relied on each other day after day, for many years. Baan was twenty-six and he had been considered a man since he was thirteen, since his initiation ceremony. This involved him being left in the savannah with four other boys with only the advice of the elders and minimal weapons to survive. This process lasted three months.

Baan remembers most of this period as frightening. He had been coming to terms with unsettling behavioural tendencies that had been programmed by millions of years of evolution. He was at the beginning of a momentous transition, changing under a fresh influx of the powerful hormone, testosterone, into a physically mature man. He was developing body hair, defined muscles, bigger shoulders, burgeoning sexuality, an appetite for risk and potentially elevated levels of aggression. This ritual, this rite of passage, would help him come to terms with these changes. It would be a clear demonstration that testosterone is at the root of what we call masculinity and the making of a man. In a more disquieting note, as writer Chip Brown notes, this initiation ceremony is also preparing him for war.

The five boys realised if they bonded together in adversity, it would help their chances of survival. As a team, they were capable of hunting and killing small animals and they knew how to search for berries, nuts and other foods. The elders had taught them from an early age how to make and transport fire, something their tribe had been doing for thousands of years. This way, they could cook their meals, keep warm at night while huddling around the embers and warn off predators.

When they returned from the adventure, they were welcomed home as men, their rites of passage acknowledged. Now they could leave the children's quarters and sleep in the men's huts. For necessity, the women lived in another part of the settlement, next to the children.

The community was not large or permanent and comprised about forty people. Basically they were nomads, following available foods as the seasons and animal migrations dictated.

There was probably a high attrition rate among the hunters – the high-risk takers, or bravest, often dying young or becoming invalided. They would sacrifice for the tribe. Extra men stepped up to fill these gaps. The other four men from Baan's initiation were now his closest and trusted friends. They formed a formidable core of the hunting group. Along with the rest of the hunters, they were not just providers – they were conditioned to protect. Fighters who, when called upon, would fiercely defend their tribe.

Baan knew most of the tribes in the region as they were often related and moved in the same traditional hunting locations. Tribes were generally not sustainable after growing to about forty to fifty members; communication and law-keeping became difficult. As a tribe expanded, generally doubling every twenty-five years or so, adventurous leaders, alpha males in our language, would move away to start their own tribe. As situations dictated, some may be less than alpha and possibly some had been rejected. As time moved on, separate languages evolved, but Baan could still understand the different dialects. These tribes shared basically the same traditions, histories, culture and belief systems. They were generally not a threat.

However, if any unfamiliar tribe, or tribesman, ventured into their territory, by accident or with ideas of occupation, Baan and his warriors' reaction was quick, powerful and often deadly. When it comes to survival, human beings, particularly those of pre-history, could be as brutal as any archaic or primordial species. Kill or be killed was essentially the law of the jungle – or the plains.

The concept of the "arms race", a pattern of competitive acquisition of military capability, kept tribes alert for developing more efficient technology, for warfare and for securing food.

The deadliest weapon was the spear. A beautifully crafted piece of hard, slick wood, two metres in length with a sharpened stone attached to the end. Baan could throw his with deadly accuracy up to fifty metres. Other men had finely made hand axes. A sharpened sliver of stone was sealed in place to a deer antler or piece of hard wood with gum cement and bindings made of strong vines.

Communication and language were elementary but effective. The men used a great deal of gesturing and variations of signs, linked to basic monosyllabic words. It was efficient, particularly when it was important to be quiet such as when stalking a prey. A simple, clear, quiet or mouthed word here and a sign there.

So alert were the hunter gatherers' basic senses, but particularly acuity of smell, that Baan could detect zebras were somewhere in the vicinity. He led the band towards where he was sure he would find them.

Suddenly Baan raised one hand, signalling the band to stop and quickly gestured ahead with the other. He had sighted a young zebra, grazing some metres away from a larger dazzle. He pointed... this would be their target. The men fanned out in a familiar circular pattern. Each knew their positions and strategy, developed from years of collaborative and successful hunting. Using the elephant grass as cover (it can grow to two or three metres), Baan was the first to move within firing range.

He signalled to the others he was ready and moved out of the grass. He stealthily approached the zebra. Startled, the zebra looked up, its eyes wide with fear. The animal spun around and began to run in the opposite direction, but was wheeled again by other emerging men. The confused animal, now in panic mode, raced straight towards Baan, who was ready. He had his spear raised, primed to throw.

Strongly and swiftly, Baan's powerful gluteal and rotator trunk muscles exploded into action, releasing the coiled-up energy. Baan's shoulder spun forward and catapulted the spear at 100 kilometres an hour. He was deadly accurate.

Baan heard a resounding thump as the spear smashed into the zebra, directly piercing its chest. The wounded beast staggered, spurting blood from the wound, then fell. Other men raced in and one, swinging a raised axe, swiftly brought the weapon down behind the zebra's skull. There was a sickening sound as the impact cracked the cervical vertebra, instantly slicing the nervous system, paralysing and killing the animal.

Other men deftly cut off the skin with sharp stones. The hide would be used for clothing and containers. Others dissected cuts of meat, offal and bones from the carcass and triumphantly headed back to the tribe. The women would continue the butchering back at the community.

The tribe would eat well for the next few days. Their regular fruit and berries diet that the women had prepared would be subsidised with meat.

As the victorious troupe entered the tribal grounds with their kill, there were many calls of goodwill and yells of encouragement. The tribe had enough basic words to allow friends to call excitedly to particular men in the group. Their language granted individuals enough communication to form personal identities, generally reflecting their status within the tribe.

Baan was always happy to return to the village. The women were mostly strong and athletic as befits a nomadic existence. They accepted their role of maintaining the village and the children with enthusiasm. One, Adira, was the mother of Baan's children. He always appreciated her femininity and protected her, aware of her soft and rounded body, expanding pelvis and breasts swelling for lactation.

Researchers acknowledge hunter-gatherers as one of the most satisfied and successful societies in history.